Study Guide to Accompany

Clinical Drug Therapy

RATIONALES FOR NURSING PRACTICE

SEVENTH EDITION

Mary Jo Kirkpatrick, MSN, RN
Assistant Professor and Director
Associate of Science in Nursing
Mississippi University for Women
Columbus, Mississippi

Anne Collins Abrams, MSN, RN
Associate Professor, Emeritus
Department of Baccalaureate and Graduate Nursing
College of Health Sciences
Eastern Kentucky University
Richmond, Kentucky

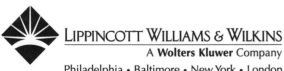

LIPPINCOTT WILLIAMS & WILKINS
A **Wolters Kluwer** Company
Philadelphia • Baltimore • New York • London
Buenos Aires • Hong Kong • Sydney • Tokyo

Acquisitions Editor: Margaret Zuccarini
Managing Editor: Doris Wray
Editorial Assistant: Carol DeVault
Production Editor: Danielle Litka
Senior Production Manager: Helen Ewan
Design Coordinator: Brett MacNaughton
Manufacturing Manager: William Alberti
Compositor: Lippincott Williams & Wilkins
Printer: Victor Graphics

Seventh Edition

9 8 7 6 5 4 3

ISBN: 0-7817-3927-6

Care has been taken to confirm the accuracy of the information presented and to
describe generally accepted practices. However, the authors, editors, and publisher
are not responsible for errors or omissions or for any consequences from application
of the information in this book and make no warranty, express or implied, with
respect to the content of the publication.

The authors, editors, and publisher have exerted every effort to ensure that drug
selection and dosage set forth in this text are in accordance with the current
recommendations and practice at the time of publication. However, in view of
ongoing research, changes in government regulations, and the constant flow of
information relating to drug therapy and drug reactions, the reader is urged to check
the package insert for each drug for any change in indications and dosage and for
added warnings and precautions. This is particularly important when the
recommended agent is a new or infrequently employed drug.

Some drugs and medical devices presented in this publication have Food and Drug
Administration (FDA) clearance for limited use in restricted research settings. It is the
responsibility of the health care provider to ascertain the FDA status of each drug or
device planned for use in his or her clinical practice.

LWW.com

Contents

CHAPTER 1

Introduction to Pharmacology

■ Exercises

Define the following.

pharmacology _____

_____

_____

biotechnology _____

_____

drug therapy_____

_____

prototypes _____

_____

_____

medications _____

_____

generic drug name _____

_____

_____

systemic drug effects_____

_____

trade drug name _____

_____

_____

synthetic chemical compounds _____

_____

_____

over-the-counter (OTC) _____

_____

_____

Answer in essay form.

1. Explain the advantages of synthetic drugs in relation to pure form drugs.

2. Discuss pharmacoeconomics.

3. Compare the two routes of access to therapeutic drugs.

4. How do you distinguish between trade names and generic names of drugs?

5. How are drugs classified?

Fill in the chart.

Name	Year	Provision
	1970	Regulated distribution of narcotics and other drugs of abuse
Durham-Humphrey		Designated drugs that are prescribed by a physician and dispensed by a pharmacist
Kefauver-Harris Amendment	1962	
	1914	Controlled the manufacture, importation, transportation, and distribution of opium, cocaine, marijuana, and their derivatives
Sherley Amendment	1912	

Match the following characteristics with the categories of controlled substances.

1. _____ may be dispensed in some states by a pharmacist without a physician's prescription

2 _____ drugs that are not approved for medical use

3. _____ drugs that are used medically and have high abuse potential

4. _____ prescription appetite suppressants except amphetamines

5. _____ abuse of drugs may lead to psychological or physical dependence

6. _____ codeine, morphine, and cocaine

7. _____ heroin, LSD, and marijuana

8. _____ commonly used sedatives and hypnotics

9. _____ drugs that contain moderate amounts of controlled substances

10. _____ drugs with some potential for abuse

a. Schedule I
b. Schedule II
c. Schedule III
d. Schedule IV
e. Schedule V

■ Review Questions

1. Which of the following deals with how drugs are used in the prevention, diagnosis, and treatment of disease?
   a. pharmacokinetics
   b. pharmacotherapy
   c. pharmacogenetics
   d. pharmacodynamics

2. Which law established official standards and requirements for accurate labeling of drugs?
   a. Pure Food and Drug Act of 1906
   b. Food, Drug and Cosmetic Act of 1938
   c. Kefauver-Harris Amendment of 1962
   d. Sherley Amendment

3. The physician has ordered phentermine, an appetite suppressant, for your client. In explaining the potential for abuse, you are aware that this drug is categorized as a:
   a. Schedule II drug
   b. Schedule III drug
   c. Schedule IV drug
   d. Schedule V drug

4. New drugs are categorized according to:
   a. half-life and bioavailability
   b. side effects and contraindications
   c. cost and availability
   d. review priority and therapeutic potential

5. Most drugs are prescribed for:
   a. local effects
   b. systemic effects
   c. immediate effects
   d. long-term effects

6. Penicillin is the standard by which other antibacterial drugs are compared and is considered a/an:
   a. regulatory drug
   b. experimental drug
   c. prototype drug
   d. placebo-controlled drug

7. Testing of new drugs usually will continue if:
   a. there are excessive side and toxic effects
   b. there is evidence of safety and therapeutic potential
   c. human subjects will participate in a clinical trial
   d. there is an increased number of people who need the drug

8. Which of the following is an advantage of using OTC drugs?
   a. self-diagnosis of an illness
   b. delay in having to seek treatment from health care provider
   c. faster and easier access to effective treatment
   d. insurance coverage for OTC drugs

9. A nurse would know that Schedule II controlled drugs:
   a. must be reordered after 6 months or five refills
   b. may be sold over the counter
   c. may be refilled once with a new prescription
   d. cannot be refilled

10. In studying pharmacology, the most important strategy is to:
    a. focus on therapeutic classifications and their prototypes
    b. memorize all drugs and their side effects
    c. not worry about the therapeutic effects
    d. use only the *Physicians' Desk Reference* as a source for drug information

■ Cell Physiology Diagram, Part I

Fill in the blanks in Figure 1-1 with the terms below.

Golgi apparatus   Cell membrane
Cytoplasm   Mitochondria
Endoplasmic reticulum   Chromatin
Nucleus   Lysosomes
Ribosomes

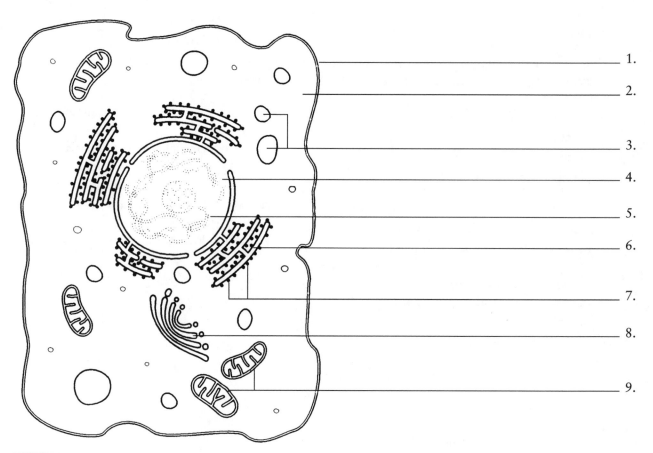

1. _____

2. _____

3. _____

4. _____

5. _____

6. _____

7. _____

8. _____

9. _____

FIGURE 1-1.

■ Cell Physiology Diagram, Part II

Answer the following.

1. Explain the relationship between the physiology of a body cell and the pharmacodynamics of a drug.

2. Examine the role of histamine and prostaglandin in the inflammatory process.

CHAPTER 2

Basic Concepts and Processes

■ Exercises

Match the following terms with their definitions.

1. ____ pharmacokinetics

2. ____ absorption

3. ____ bioavailability

4. ____ distribution

5. ____ metabolism

6. ____ excretion

7. ____ half-life

8. ____ pharmacodynamics

9. ____ receptors

10. ____ agonists

11. ____ antagonists

12. ____ synergism

13. ____ placebo

14. ____ drug tolerance

15. ____ idiosyncracy

a. Drugs that inhibit cell function

b. Unexpected reaction to a drug that occurs the first time it is given

c. Involves drug movement through the body to sites of action

d. The portion of a dose that reaches the systemic circulation and is available to act on body cells

e. The method by which drugs are inactivated or detoxified by the body

f. Refers to elimination of a drug from the body

g. Drugs that produce effects similar to those produced by naturally occurring substances

h. When two drugs with different sites or mechanisms of action produce greater effects when taken together than does either dose when taken alone

i. The process that occurs between the time a drug enters the body and the time it enters the bloodstream to be circulated

j. Occurs when the body becomes accustomed to a drug over time so that a larger dose is required to produce the same effect

k. Involves the transport of drug molecules within the body

l. The time required for the blood concentration of a drug to decrease by 50%

m. Involves drug actions on target cells

n. A pharmacologically inactive substance

o. Proteins located within cells

Answer the following.

1. List factors influencing drug action.

2. List the mechanisms that can cause drug fever.

3. List goals of treatment for a poisoned client.

4. List the components of protoplasm.

5. List the three main pathways of drug movement across cell membranes.

Define the following.

passive diffusion _____

_____

_____

facilitated diffusion _____

_____

_____

active transport _____

_____

_____

Fill in the chart.

Drug	Antidote
heparin	
	naloxone (Narcan)
	diphenhydramine HCL (Benadryl)
warfarin (Coumadin)	
	acetylcysteine (Mucomyst)
beta blockers	

■ Review Questions

1. When caring for the elderly, the nurse is aware that the effect of aging on the liver results in:
   a. reduced intensity of drug effects
   b. reduced incidence of toxicity
   c. prolonged drug effects
   d. inadequate blood levels of a drug

2. Vistaril, given in combination with Talwin, counteracts the side effects of nausea caused by the Talwin. The drug–drug interaction responsible for the desired effect is:
   a. addition
   b. antagonism
   c. synergism
   d. potentiation

3. On the 2 AM round, the nurse finds a client restless and unable to sleep. A sedative-hypnotic is administered. Two hours later, the nurse finds the client irritable and restless. This is characteristic of:
   a. an allergic reaction
   b. a teratogenic effect
   c. a tachyphalactic reaction
   d. an idiosyncratic response

4. A client is receiving an antibiotic for an infection. The nurse teaches the client that taking most drugs with food will:
   a. have no effect on the physiological action of the drug
   b. increase the rate of absorption of the drug
   c. decrease the amount of drug being absorbed
   d. increase appetite

5. Which cell structure is called the "manager" of cellular activities?
   a. Golgi complex
   b. mitrochondria
   c. cytoplasm
   d. nucleus

6. Thyroid disorders mostly affect which pharmacokinetic function?
   a. absorption
   b. distribution
   c. metabolism
   d. excretion

7. Which of the following clients will a nurse expect to experience alterations in drug metabolism?

    a. a 52-year-old male with cirrhosis of the liver

    b. a 35-year-old female with ulcerative colitis

    c. a 41-year-old male with cancer of the stomach

    d. a 60-year-old female with acute renal failure

8. Your client has been taking a medication for several months for chronic back pain. He tells you that the medication is no longer relieving the pain. In discussing this with the client, you explain the possibility of:

    a. drug fever

    b. diffusion

    c. drug tolerance

    d. hypersensitivity

9. The process of the movement of a drug from the place it enters the body until it reaches the circulation is which of the following pharmacokinetic activities?

    a. absorption

    b. distribution

    c. metabolism

    d. excretion

10. The amount of a drug that gets into the circulation and is available to the tissues is referred to as:

    a. bioavailability

    b. cumulative toxicity

    c. serum half-life

    d. detoxification

Administering Medications

■ Exercises

Answer the following.

1. Define the "five rights."

2. Explain why the nurse is legally responsible for safe and accurate administration of medication.

3. List all the components of a medication order.

4. Define the term *parenteral*.

5. Explain why controlled-release tablets and capsules should never be broken or crushed.

Place a T (true) or F (false) in each blank.

1. _____ A nurse should never question a physician if a drug order is unclear.

2. _____ When calculating a child's drug dosage, always ask a pharmacist or another nurse to do the calculation also and compare the results.

3. _____ All nurse practitioners are allowed to prescribe medications.

4. _____ A nurse is not legally responsible for actions delegated to other health care personnel.

5. _____ Only the nurse is responsible for getting medication to a client.

6. _____ Unit dose wrappings of oral drugs should be left with the medication until the nurse is in the presence of the client and is ready to administer the drug.

7. _____ Nurses may take verbal or telephone orders from physicians.

8. _____ Some drugs are available in one dosage form only.

9. _____ Enteric-coated tablets delay absorption until the medication reaches the stomach.

10. _____ The metric system is the most commonly used system of measurement.

11. _____ Units express the ionic activity of a drug.

12. _____ Single-dose vials contain preservatives and should be kept for other dosages after initial use.

13. ____ The term *gauge* refers to the lumen size of the needle.

14. ____ A 22-gauge 1½ inch needle is used for subcutaneous injections.

15. ____ The most convenient route of drug administration is the oral route.

Match the abbreviations with the appropriate terms.

1. ____ cubic centimeter   a. OS
2. ____ before meals   b. PRN
3. ____ right eye   c. pc
4. ____ by mouth   d. qd
5. ____ drops   e. PO
6. ____ immediately   f. q 4h
7. ____ when needed   g. cc
8. ____ after meals   h. ad lib
9. ____ daily   i. stat
10. ____ every 4 hours   j. OD
11. ____ left eye   k. hs
12. ____ bedtime   l. bid
13. ____ twice daily   m. ac
14. ____ as desired   n. qid
15. ____ four times daily   o. gtt

Fill in the blank with the approximate equivalent.

1. 1 kg = _____ lb
2. 1 g = _____mg
3. 60 mg = _____gr
4. 1 mL = _____ cc
5. 1 cc = _____ minims
6. 1 cup = _____ mL
7. 1 mg = _____mcg
8. 30 mg = _____oz

9. 1 dram = _____mL
10. 15 gtt = _____ mL

Convert each item to the equivalent.

1. 30 drops = ____minims
2. 50 lbs = ____kg
3. 2 drams = ____mL
4. 3500 mg = ____g
5. 2.5 tsp = ____mL
6. 15 mL = ____cc
7. 2 L = ____mL
8. 32 minims = ____cc
9. 500 mL = ____cups
10. 2.5 mg = ____mcg

Calculate the following drug dosages.

1. Order: Tegretol 800 mg/d
   Label: Tegretol XL 200 mg/tablet
   How many tablets will the client take each day?

2. Order: Benadryl elixir 25 mg
   Label: Benadryl elixir 12.5 mg per 5 mL

3. Order: KCL 40 mEq PO
   Label: KCL 10 mEq/15 mL

4. Order: Heparin 1500 units IV
   Label: Heparin 1000 units/mL

5. Order: Synthroid 50 mcg PO daily
   Label: Synthroid 0.025 mg/tablet

6. Robitussin cough syrup 600 mg in 1 oz is available. The order is for 225 mg. How many cc should you administer?

7. Keflex is available in 250-mg capsules. Keflex 0.5 gm PO is ordered. How many capsules should you administer?

8. Prepare penicillin 600,000 units IM. Penicillin 1,200,000 units/mL is available. How many mL will you administer?

9. Demerol 50 mg/mL is available. The order is for Demerol 100 mg. How many mL will you administer?

10. Maalox 1/2 oz is ordered. How many cc would you administer?

■ Review Questions

1. The client is to receive ampicillin 500 mg PO tid ac. Which of the following reflects proper scheduling?
   a. 4 AM, 12 noon, 8 PM
   b. 7 AM, 11 AM, 6 PM
   c. 7 AM, 1 PM, 8 PM
   d. 8 AM, 12 noon, 4 PM, 8 PM

2. A client asks the nurse whether he can divide his enteric-coated tablet in half. The nurse tells him not to because dividing the drug will:
   a. make the drug less potent
   b. cause severe abdominal cramps
   c. alter the drug's absorption
   d. produce no therapeutic effect

3. The client is a 4-year-old who has a temperature of 103° and is vomiting. The physician has ordered Tylenol for the fever. The nurse would administer the Tylenol in which of the following forms?
   a. liquid
   b. lozenge
   c. tablet
   d. suppository

4. The nurse is assigned to administer medication to 10 clients. Which of the following would be the initial action of the nurse before preparing the medications?
   a. Identify the client by asking him what his name is.
   b. Wash his hands.
   c. Explain the action of the medications to the client.
   d. Record the administration of the medication.

5. Which of the following statements best describes the reason for aspiration before injecting medication into a muscle?

   a. to determine whether the needle is in the correct muscle

   b. to decrease discomfort

   c. to avoid major nerves in the area

   d. to avoid injecting the medication into a blood vessel

6. The client is 15 months old and is hospitalized for pneumonia. The nurse will administer an intramuscular injection in which of the following muscles?

   a. deltoid

   b. dorsogluteal muscle

   c. ventrogluteal muscle

   d. vastus lateralis

7. The term for IV administration of a drug over 15 to 60 minutes is called:

   a. a loading dose

   b. an IVP (push)

   c. a peripheral IV infusion

   d. an IVPB (piggyback)

8. Which of the following is proper placement of the needle for an intramuscular injection into the dorsogluteal site?

   a. below the greater trochanter and posterior iliac spine

   b. above and inside a diagonal line drawn from the greater trochanter of the femur to the anterior superior iliac crest

   c. below the anterior superior iliac spine and above the greater trochanter

   d. above and outside a diagonal line drawn from the greater trochanter of the femur to the posterior superior iliac spine

9. Which of the following is true regarding administration of medications by the oral route?

   a. It is convenient and relatively inexpensive.

   b. Oral administration is best for all clients.

   c. Gastrointestinal upset rarely occurs.

   d. Water given with medication retards drug absorption.

10. The nurse is to administer gentamicin gtt 2 OD. The nurse will administer the drug in the client's:

    a. right eye

    b. left eye

    c. right ear

    d. left ear

■ Subcutaneous Injections Diagram

Mark on Figure 3-1 where subcutaneous injections can be administered.

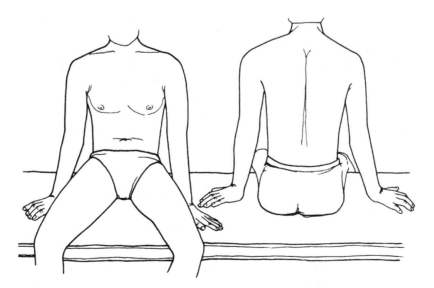

FIGURE 3-1.

CHAPTER 4

Nursing Process in Drug Therapy

■ Exercises

Fill in the blank.

1. The _____·_____ is a systematic method used to gather data to plan and implement client care and evaluate the outcomes of that care.

2. Nurses plan and provide client care based on _____ data.

3. Client goals should be stated in terms of _____ behavior.

4. _____ can be evaluated soon after drug administration or after longer periods of time.

5. _____ _____ are guidelines for client care with specific conditions.

Answer the following.

1. Give an example of a nursing diagnosis related to drug therapy.

2. List three examples of expected outcomes related to prescribed drug therapy.

3. List five areas of nursing intervention in relation to drug therapy.

4. List five examples of interventions that decrease the need for drug therapy.

5. Explain why client teaching related to drug therapy is important.

6. Why do nurses have difficulties in evaluating outcomes of drug therapy?

7. List major components of critical paths.

8. Discuss current legislation in regard to herbal and dietary supplements.

9. What are the two major concerns that health care providers have concerning the use of herbal and dietary supplements?

10. What must be considered in pediatric drug therapy?

Place a T (true) or F (false) in each blank.

1. ____ The goal of drug therapy should be to minimize beneficial effects and maximize adverse effects.

2. ____ Drugs should not be prescribed for conditions for which nondrug measures are effective.

3. ____ Few variables influence a drug's effect on the body.

4. ____ Decreasing the number of drugs and the frequency of administration increases the client's compliance with prescribed drugs.

5. ____ Fixed-dose drug combinations are commonly used.

6. ____ The smallest amount of the most potent drug for therapeutic benefit should be given.

7. ____ Clients with severe kidney disease often need smaller doses of drugs that are excreted by the kidneys.

8. ____ A physician may order a loading dose of a drug if it has a short half-life.

9. ____ Drug therapy is less predictable in children than in adults.

10. ____ Older adults are usually less likely to metabolize and excrete drugs efficiently.

11. ____ For elderly clients receiving long-term drug therapy at home, childproof containers should be avoided.

12. ____ Liver impairment does not interfere with drug metabolism.

13. ____ Alcohol is toxic to the liver and increases the risk of hepatotoxicity.

14. ____ The dosage should be reduced for drugs that are extensively metabolized in the liver because toxicity can occur in clients with hepatic disease.

15. ____ For a critically ill client, therapeutic drug effects may be increased.

Match uses to herbal and dietary supplements. Some uses may be used more than once.

1. ____ chamomile

2. ____ feverfew

3. ____ ginkgo biloba

4. ____ garlic

5. ____ echinacea

6. ____ ginseng

7. ____ glucosamine

8. ____ black cohosh

9. ____ chondroitin

10. ____ ephedra

11. ____ Saint John's wort

12. ____ saw palmetto

13. ____ melatonin

14. ____ valerian

15. ____ kava

a. Weight loss

b. Arthritis

c. Insomnia

d. Depression

e. Abdominal cramping

f. High cholesterol

g. Menopausal symptoms

h. Stamina and strength

i. Urinary symptoms

j. Common cold

k. Anxiety and stress

l. Memory

m. Migraines

■ Clinical Challenge

Your 88-year-old client is being discharged from the hospital with a newly prescribed drug. Formulate a topical outline for a teaching plan you would use in this clinical situation.

■ Review Questions

1. A client is being discharged on an antibiotic and has very little knowledge concerning the drug. Which of the following best reflects an expected goal of client-teaching related to the antibiotic?

   a. Client will be able to interpret culture and sensitivity test.

   b. Family members will understand the physiological action of the antibiotic.

   c. Client will exercise three times a week.

   d. Client will be able to identify two adverse effects of the antibiotic.

2. A 62-year-old client has just been diagnosed as having diabetes mellitus. Before giving him any medication, the nurse must first assess all of the following except:

    a. medications taken at home

    b. other medical conditions that may interfere with drug therapy for the diabetes mellitus

    c. medication allergies

    d. his response to the new medication

3. A client is in the cardiac care unit following a mild cardiac infarction. She is on multiple drug therapy, including three intramuscular (IM) injections per day. Which of the following would be the appropriate nursing diagnosis related to the administration of the IM injections?

    a. altered nutrition: more than body requirements related to overeating

    b. anxiety related to three IM injections each day

    c. impaired social interaction related to being in the cardiac care unit

    d. noncompliance related to overuse of medication

4. Which statement by the client with heart disease would indicate that health teaching related to medication was ineffective?

    a. "It's best to take my medication as the doctor ordered."

    b. "It shouldn't matter that I skip a couple of doses now and then."

    c. "I will call the clinic if I experience any side effects from my medications."

    d. "I will get all of my medications at the same pharmacy."

5. During drug therapy, clients with liver disease are monitored for which of the following?

    a. dizziness

    b. jaundice

    c. headache

    d. constipation

6. The goal of drug therapy in critically ill clients is to:

    a. support vital functions

    b. decrease medication use

    c. disregard laboratory tests related to the client's physiological condition

    d. increase or decrease dietary intake, depending on weight of the client

7. Which of the following herbal/dietary supplements could increase the potential for bleeding when taking aspirin?

    a. melatonin

    b. saw palmetto

    c. ginseng

    d. chondroitin

8. When implementing medication therapy for a client, the nurse is responsible for which of the following actions?

    a. changing the drug dosage if side effects occur

    b. discontinuing the drug if the client does not want to take it

    c. sharing information concerning therapeutic value of the drug in other clients

    d. checking for the correct dosage of the drug prior to administration

9. Which phase of the nursing process requires the nurse to formulate a client outcome related to the administration of medication?

    a. assessment

    b. planning

    c. implementation

    d. evaluation

10. In gathering assessment data from a medication history, which of the following would be most helpful to the nurse in planning client care?

    a. the name of the pharmacist the client talks to regarding his medication

    b. a list of all prescribed and over-the-counter medications and herbal and dietary supplements the client takes

    c. the medication history of the client's mother

    d. dietary intake for 1 day

CHAPTER 5

Physiology of the Central Nervous System

■ Exercises

Match the following with its characteristics.

1. _____ synapse
2. _____ myelin cover
3. _____ gamma-aminobutyric acid (GABA)
4. _____ serotonin
5. _____ receptors
6. _____ glutamate
7. _____ dopamine
8. _____ amino acids
9. _____ acetylcholine
10. _____ neurotransmitters

a. Protects and insulates the axon
b. Chemical substances that send messages from one neuron to another
c. Proteins embedded in the cell membranes of neurons
d. A precursor substance in the synthesis of norepinephrine
e. Neurotransmitter in the cholinergic system located in the motor cortex and basal ganglia
f. The small gap between neurons in a chain
g. Thought to produce sleep by inhibiting central nervous system (CNS) activity and arousal
h. Important neurotransmitter in the CNS that may be involved in the pathogenesis of epilepsy
i. Major inhibitory transmitter in the CNS
j. Can serve as structural components for protein synthesis and transmitters

Fill in the blank.

1. Drugs affecting the CNS are classified as either _____ or _____.
2. The _____ _____ is a pathway from the brain to the peripheral nervous system.
3. The CNS is comprised mainly of two types of cells, which are the _____ and the _____.
4. Three main types of neurotransmitters are _____ _____, _____, and _____.
5. _____ _____ are necessary for neurotransmitter release from storage sites.
6. Neurons are composed of a _____ _____, a _____, and an _____.
7. Synapses may be either _____ or _____.
8. An _____ is a fingerlike projection that causes impulses away from the cell body.
9. _____ is found in large amounts in the hypothalamus and the limbic system.
10. The _____ receives impulses related to sensations, such as heat, cold, and pain.

Answer the following.

1. List characteristics of CNS depression.

2. List characteristics of CNS stimulation.

3. Explain characteristics that allow neurons to communicate with other cells.

4. List three mechanisms by which free neurotransmitter molecules are removed from the synapse.

5. List four factors that affect the availability and function of neurotransmitters.

■ Review Questions

1. The area of the brain responsible for helping maintain homeostasis is the:
   a. cerebellum
   b. limbic system
   c. cerebrum
   d. hypothalamus

2. Normal function of skeletal muscle is influenced by:
   a. acetylcholine
   b. dopamine
   c. glutamate
   d. serotonin

3. Your client has Alzheimer's disease. You are aware that in this condition there is decrease in:
   a. acetylcholine
   b. aspartate

   c. serotonin
   d. glycine

4. Neurons that carry messages to the central nervous system are called:
   a. efferent neurons
   b. glia neurons
   c. afferent neurons
   d. motor neurons

5. Which of the following is an energy source for brain cells?
   a. thiamine
   b. glucose
   c. oxygen
   d. oxytocin

6. Your client has had a cerebrovascular accident (CVA, or stroke) and is having difficulty in speaking. You are aware that, most likely, the CVA involved which of the following areas in the brain?
   a. cerebral cortex
   b. thalamus
   c. hypothalamus
   d. medulla oblongata

7. Your client is experiencing CNS depression. Which of the following would you observe in your client?
   a. increased muscle tone
   b. hyperactive reflexes
   c. short attention span
   d. increased perception of cold sensations

8. Which of the following plays an important role in blood coagulation?
   a. tryptophan
   b. glycine
   c. aspartate
   d. serotonin

9. The hypothalamus regulates the production of oxytocin, which:
   a. regulates body temperature
   b. initiates uterine contractions
   c. regulates arterial blood pressure
   d. decides which impulses to transmit to the cerebral cortex

10. Your client has a head injury. The physician explains that most of the trauma was located in the cerebellum area of the brain. You would expect your client to:

    a. have a hard time maintaining balance and posture

    b. exhibit rigidity and increased muscle tone

    c. exhibit decreased mental alertness

    d. have frequent periods of crying

■ Neurotransmission Diagram, Part I

Fill in the blanks in Figure 5-1 with the terms below.

Receptor sites
Neurotransmitters
Presynaptic nerve terminal
Presynaptic nerve cell membrane
Postsynaptic nerve terminal
Synapse
Release site
Postsynaptic nerve cell membrane

■ Neurotransmission Diagram, Part II

Complete the following sentences.

1. Norepinephrine is an excitatory neurotransmitter that affects mood and motor activity after crossing the _____ from the postganglionic sympathetic nervous system neurons and binding to _____ in the postsynaptic nerve cell membrane of the nerves that supply blood vessels to the adrenal medulla.

2. Acetylcholine is an inhibitory neurotransmitter that exerts inhibitory effects on organs supplied by the vagus nerves by binding at _____.

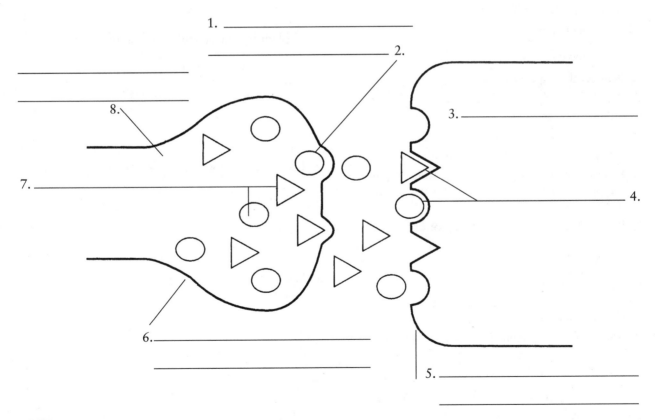

1. _____
2. _____
8. _____
7. _____
3. _____
4. _____
6. _____
5. _____

FIGURE 5-1.

CHAPTER 6

Opioid Analgesics and Opioid Antagonists

■ Exercises

Match the following.

1. _____ thalamus

2. _____ patient-controlled analgesia

3. _____ nociceptors

4. _____ visceral pain

5. _____ opioid peptides

6. _____ chronic pain

7. _____ bradykinin

8. _____ neuropathic pain

9. _____ acute pain

10. _____ somatic pain

a. Pain-producing substance

b. Pain originating from abdominal and thoracic organs

c. Pain lasting 3 to 6 months

d. Relay station for incoming stimuli

e. Pain originating from injury of peripheral pain receptors, nerves, or the central nervous system (CNS)

f. Pain described as sharp, lancing, or cutting

g. Interact with opiate receptors to inhibit pain transmission

h. Free nerve endings

i. Pain originating in structural tissues, such as bone, muscle, and soft tissue

j. Allows for self-administration of medication

Answer the following.

1. Describe the process that must occur for a person to feel pain.

2. How is pain classified?

3. Explain the physiological action of an opioid analgesic.

4. List pharmacological effects of opioid analgesics.

5. Why would opioid analgesics be contraindicated in a client with chronic lung disease?

6. Explain how opioid agonists/antagonists work in the body.

7. Describe the physiological action of opioid antagonists.

8. Explain the concept of morphine as a "nonceiling" drug.

9. Why does a dose of an oral opioid analgesic need to be larger than an injected dose?

10. List characteristics of opiate withdrawal.

Place a T (true) or F (false) in each blank.

1. ____ Opioid antagonists reverse respiratory depression caused by all CNS depressants.

2. ____ Morphine (Tagamet), given in combination with cimetidine, may increase CNS and respiratory depression.

3. ____ An opioid analgesic, given in combination with an antihypertensive drug, may cause hypertension.

4. ____ Clients taking naltrexone (ReVia) do not respond to opioid analgesics if pain control is needed.

5. ____ The drug of choice in treatment of opioid overdose is naloxone (Narcan).

6. ____ The usual dose of codeine for cough is 50 to 60 mg q 4h PRN.

7. ____ Crushing or chewing a long-acting tablet of an opioid analgesic delays the release of the drug.

8. ____ Referred pain is pain occurring from tissue damage in one area of the body but felt in another area.

9. ____ Opioid analgesics are not indicated for long-term use in chronic pain associated with osteoarthritis.

10. ____ Opioid analgesics are commonly used to manage pain associated with disease processes and invasive diagnostic and therapeutic procedures.

■ Clinical Challenge

Discuss the difference in pain management in a client in acute pain who is 1 day post-operative from hip replacement surgery and a client who is experiencing chronic cancer pain.

■ Review Questions

1. It may be necessary to repeat doses of naloxone (Narcan) to a client who has had too much morphine because the opioid antagonist:
   a. has less strength in each dose than do individual doses of morphine
   b. has a shorter half-life than does morphine
   c. combined with morphine, increases the physiological action of the morphine
   d. causes the respiratory rate to decrease

2. Which of the following would indicate a therapeutic effect of an opioid analgesic for a client who has been experiencing severe pain?

   a. restlessness during the night hours

   b. increased participation in AM care activities

   c. shorter intervals between medication administration

   d. increased facial grimacing during movement

3. Before administering an opioid analgesic, the initial action of the nurse would be to:

   a. check the apical pulse and compare it with the radial pulse

   b. check the blood pressure lying and standing

   c. check the temperature

   d. check the rate, depth, and rhythm of respirations

4. It's Friday night, and you are working in the emergency department. Your first client is a 17-year-old high school soccer player who is complaining of severe muscle spasms in her left leg. You would classify her pain as:

   a. acute pain

   b. chronic pain

   c. neuropathic pain

   d. somatic pain

5. Your post-op client will be receiving hydromorphone (Dilaudid) via patient-controlled analgesia (PCA) and is having second thoughts about administering his own medication for fear of overdosing himself. A nursing diagnosis for your client would be:

   a. knowledge deficient related to the use of PCA

   b. impaired gas exchange related to the surgery

   c. anxiety related to surgical procedure

   d. impaired judgment related to increased dosage of medication

6. Your client is to receive propoxyphene (Darvon) as needed for pain. Which of the following would be an appropriate medication order for your client?

   a. 390 mg qid IM

   b. 65 mg q 4h PRN PO

   c. 65 mg bid PRN PO

   d. 100 mg q 2h PO

7. You have just administered an IM injection of meperidine (Demerol) to your client. The most important nursing measure you should perform before leaving the room should be to:

   a. close the draperies

   b. make sure the side rails are up

   c. ask all the visitors to leave the room

   d. offer your client something to drink

8. A common side effect of an opioid analgesic is:

   a. constipation

   b. diarrhea

   c. increased respirations

   d. fine hand tremors

9. You suspect that the neonate you will be receiving in the newborn intensive care unit may be experiencing opioid withdrawal. You will most likely see signs and symptoms that include:

   a. tremors

   b. decreased muscle tone

   c. constipation

   d. bradycardia

10. An automatic "stop order" for opioids is usually between:

    a. 24 and 36 hours

    b. 48 and 72 hours

    c. 60 and 96 hours

    d. 72 and 130 hours

Analgesic-Antipyretic-Anti-inflammatory and Related Drugs

■ Exercises

Match the following terms with their definitions.

1. ____ pyrogens
2. ____ chondroitin
3. ____ tinnitus
4. ____ prostaglandins
5. ____ osteoarthritis
6. ____ glucosamine
7. ____ rheumatoid arthritis
8. ____ Reye's syndrome
9. ____ inflammation
10. ____ bursitis

a. Normal body response to tissue damage
b. Inflammation of a cavity in connective tissue that contains synovial fluid
c. Normal component of joint cartilage
d. Chemical mediators found in most body tissue
e. Ringing or roaring in the ears
f. A disease that affects the cartilage of weight-bearing joints
g. Essential structural component of joint connective tissue
h. A chronic, painful, inflammatory disorder that affects joints and has systemic effects
i. Fever-producing agent
j. A disease seen in children under 15 associated with use of aspirin

Place a T (true) or F (false) in each blank.

1. ____ The first drug of choice for a moderate to severe migraine attack is ergotamine tartrate/caffeine (Cafergot).

2. ____ When allopurinol (Zyloprim) is taken for gout, uric acid blood levels decrease to normal range within 1 to 3 weeks.

3. ____ You must take acetaminophen with food.

4. ____ If one non-steroid anti-inflammatory drug (NSAID) is not effective, another one may produce therapeutic effects.

5. ____ Over-the-counter (OTC) ibuprofen is the same medication as prescription Motrin.

6. ____ Anticoagulants decrease the effects of indomethacin (Indocin).

7. ____ Symptoms of ergot poisoning include coolness, numbness and tingling of extremities, vomiting, and dizziness.

8. ____ Celecoxib (Celebrex) should be taken with food.

9. ____ Aspirin toxicity occurs at levels above 500 mcg/mL.

10. ____ In older adults, long-term use of NSAIDs can increase the risk of serious gastrointestinal bleeding.

Match the name with the following generic drug.

1. ____ celecoxib
2. ____ etodolac
3. ____ nabumetone
4. ____ naproxen sodium
5. ____ sulindac
6. ____ sumatriptan
7. ____ acetaminophen

8. ____ allopurinol

9. ____ ibuprofen

10. ____ rofecoxib

a. Motrin

b. Vioxx

c. Tylenol

d. Zyloprim

e. Lodine

f. Anaprox

g. Imitrex

h. Celebrex

i. Clinoril

j. Relafen

■ Clinical Challenge

Your client is brought into the emergency department complaining of nausea, vomiting, fever, tinnitus, and blurred vision. During your initial assessment, you determine that the client is mildly confused. You are aware that he has rheumatoid arthritis. What do you think his medical diagnosis will be? What would be your plan of care?

■ Review Questions

1. Your client is 9 years old and has symptoms of influenza. Her mother explains that her fever has been between 102° and 103° for the last 2 days. Which medication would you suggest be given to her?

   a. acetaminophen

   b. aspirin

   c. naproxen

   d. nabumetone

2. Your client has been diagnosed with rheumatoid arthritis. He has been placed on celecoxib (Celebrex) 100 mg tid. You will provide your client with the following information about this drug:

   a. Expect heart palpitations to occur.

   b. Take with food to decrease gastric irritation.

   c. Increase the dosage if prescribed dosage does not provide relief.

   d. Wear sunscreen when outside, due to hypersensitivity effect.

3. The emergency department nurse is expecting a client to be brought in who is exhibiting signs and symptoms of acetaminophen poisoning. The nurse will have the following drug available for administration when the client arrives:

   a. oxaprozin (Daypro)

   b. vitamin K

   c. acetylcysteine (Mucomyst)

   d. naloxone (Narcan)

4. Your client has been on naproxen (Naprosyn) for some time. When evaluating him on his return visits to the clinic, you will monitor which of the following?

   a. low-density lipoprotein

   b. serum amylase level

   c. blood glucose level

   d. bleeding time

5. Your client is to begin colchicine therapy for acute gout. You inform him that, with oral therapy, he should have pain relief within:

   a. 2 to 4 hours

   b. 6 to 12 hours

   c. 12 to 20 hours

   d. 24 to 48 hours

6. Your client has a history of migraines. She has just been given a prescription for sumatriptan (Imitrex). Which symptoms would you tell her to report to her physician immediately?

   a. decreased appetite

   b. chest pain

   c. slight weight gain

   d. fatigue

7. Which of the following statements by your client reveals a potential problem with NSAID therapy?

    a. "I take my medication with a full glass of water."

    b. "I can still have my glass of wine every night."

    c. "I should make sure my doctor checks for blood in my stool."

    d. "I have problems with swallowing, but I do not crush my tablets."

8. Your client is on an antigout drug. Your teaching plan concerning this drug in preventing the formation of uric acid kidney stones would involve which of the following?

    a. Walk at least 2 miles three times a week.

    b. Take on an empty stomach.

    c. Avoid exposure to sunlight.

    d. Drink 2 to 3 quarts of water daily.

9. A 72-year-old man has been taking a baby aspirin every day for the last 5 years. He is scheduled for major dental work in 1 month. It will be important for this man to:

    a. double the amount of aspirin he is taking

    b. avoid aspirin for 2 weeks prior to the dental procedure

    c. increase his fluid intake by 1000 cc per day 1 week prior to the dental work

    d. expect complications following the dental work

10. Your 65-year-old client has been diagnosed with osteoarthritis of the hands and feet. She reveals to you that she is having difficulty performing light housework. Which of the following would be an appropriate nursing diagnosis related to her complaint?

    a. risk for injury related to adverse drug effects

    b. activity intolerance related to pain

    c. knowledge deficient related to medical diagnosis

    d. altered nutrition related to medication

CHAPTER 8

Antianxiety and Sedative-Hypnotic Drugs

■ Exercises

Match the following terms with their definitions.

1. ____ sedative

2. ____ alprazolam (Xanax)

3. ____ kava

4. ____ midazolam (Versed)

5. ____ hypnotic

6. ____ sertraline (Zoloft)

7. ____ flumazenil

8. ____ zaleplon (Sonata)

9. ____ diazepam (Valium)

10. ____ chlordiazepoxide (Librium)

a. Herbal/dietary supplement that suppresses emotional excitability

b. Antidote for benzodiazepines

c. Prototype benzodiazepine

d. Produces sleep

e. Prescribed for obsessive-compulsive disorder

f. An oral nonbenzodiazepine schedule IV controlled substance used for short-term treatment of insomnia

g. Prescribed in acute alcohol withdrawal

h. Promotes relaxation

i. Preoperative sedation used for short-term treatment of anxiety

j. Benzodiazepine used for panic disorder

Answer the following.

1. Why is buspirone preferred over a benzodiazepine?

2. Explain the pharmacokinetics of benzodiazepines.

3. List contraindications to benzodiazepines.

4. Compare buspirone and benzodiazepines.

5. What is the goal for treatment for insomnia?

Place the generic name in the blank next to the trade name.

1. Librium _____

2. Ambien _____

3. Versed _____

4. BuSpar _____

5. Vistaril _____

6. Xanax _____

7. Sonata _____

8. Zoloft _____

9. Ativan _____

10. Restoril _____

Place T (true) or F (false) in each blank.

1. ____ Midazolam (Versed) may be mixed in the same syringe with morphine sulfate.

2. ____ At bedtime, food should be taken with zolpidem (Ambien).

3. ____ Cimetidine (Tagamet) decreases the effects of zaleplon (Sonata).

4. ____ Opioid analgesics increase effects of antianxiety and sedative-hypnotic drugs.

5. ____ Diazepam (Valium) is physically incompatible with other drugs.

6. ____ Benzodiazepines can be given intramuscularly in the deltoid muscle.

7. ____ Adverse effects of antianxiety and sedative-hypnotic drugs are caused by central nervous system depression.

8. ____ Excessive drowsiness is more likely to occur when drug therapy begins.

9. ____ Lorazepam (Ativan) is probably the benzodiazepine of first choice.

10. ____ To prevent withdrawal symptoms, benzodiazepines should be tapered in dose and gradually discontinued.

■ Clinical Challenge

Your client has been taking a benzodiazepine for 4 months. During his most recent clinic visit, you suspect that he has stopped taking the drug. What symptoms would you assess for? What would you tell him regarding discontinuing the drug?

■ Review Questions

1. Your client describes having feelings of fear and impending doom. She states that she has palpitations, shortness of breath, and sometimes dizziness and nausea. Your assessment indicates that she is having panic attacks. The most appropriate drug for your client is:
   a. hydroxyzine (Vistaril)
   b. buspirone (BuSpar)
   c. alprazolam (Xanax)
   d. lorazepam (Ativan)

2. Which of the following statements by your client indicates his understanding of his new drug, buspirone (BuSpar)?
   a. "My muscles are so relaxed after I take my medication."
   b. "BuSpar will cause me to go to sleep after I take each dose."
   c. "BuSpar gave me immediate relief the first day I took it."
   d. "It will probably take 3 to 4 weeks for my new medication to make me feel better."

3. Which of the following nondrug measures would you implement to enhance the effectiveness of an antianxiety drug?
   a. Turn out bright lights and decrease the temperature.
   b. Do not worry your client with details concerning his care.
   c. Spend at least 30 minutes explaining how his antianxiety drug will decrease his anxiety.
   d. Withhold all other medications.

4. Your client is drowsy, and his speech is slurred. He appears to have difficulty concentrating. You suspect that he is experiencing:
   a. a panic attack
   b. sleep deprivation
   c. obsessive-compulsive disorder
   d. hyperactivity

5. Which of the following drugs will decrease the effects of an antianxiety agent?
   a. nicotine
   b. alcohol
   c. cimetidine
   d. oral contraceptives

6. Your client is to receive a hypnotic for the first time. You will tell her to expect drowsiness within:
    a. 10 minutes
    b. 15 minutes
    c. 30 minutes
    d. 60 minutes

7. Which of the following is not a side effect of an antianxiety medication?
    a. hypertension
    b. hypotension
    c. confusion
    d. impaired mobility

8. When administering a sedative, you encourage your client to drink a full glass of water. When he questions you about the amount of water, the most appropriate response would be:
    a. "The water is necessary to dilute the drug."
    b. "The water increases dissolution and absorption of the drug for a faster onset of action."

c. "The more fluid you drink, the faster the elimination of the drug from the body."
d. "The fluid helps decrease the irritation to the body tissues."

9. If a client is excessively sedated at the time of the next sedative dose, you should:
    a. omit the dose and record the reason
    b. withhold the dose for 30 minutes
    c. administer flumazenil
    d. have the physician discontinue the drug

10. Your client has cirrhosis. Which of the following antianxiety agents would be appropriate for her?
    a. temazepam (Restoril)
    b. lorazepam (Ativan)
    c. buspirone (BuSpar)
    d. zaleplon (Sonata)

CHAPTER 9

Antipsychotic Drugs

■Exercises

Place T (true) or F (false) in each blank.

1. ____ Increased salivation is a common side effect of antipsychotic drugs.

2. ____ Antacids should not be taken with antipsychotic drugs.

3. ____ Most adverse effects are less likely to occur or be severe with the newer "atypical" drugs than with phenothiazines.

4. ____ Delusions indicate severe mental illness.

5. ____ Overt psychotic symptoms must be present for at least 12 months before a diagnosis of schizophrenia can be made.

6. ____ Symptoms of schizophrenia may begin gradually or suddenly.

7. ____ Overactivity of dopamine accounts for negative symptoms of schizophrenia.

8. ____ Chlorpromazine (Thorazine) was the first drug to treat psychotic disorders effectively.

9. ____ Phenothiazines may cause psychological dependence but do not cause physical dependence.

10. ____ "Atypical" antipsychotic drugs have become the first drug of choice.

Answer the following.

1. List positive symptoms of schizophrenia.

2. List negative symptoms of schizophrenia.

3. Describe the difference between "typical" antipsychotics and "atypical" antipsychotics.

4. List clinical indications for phenothiazines, other than psychiatric illnesses.

5. Why is clozapine (Clozaril) considered a second-line drug?

Fill in the blank.

1. _____ may cause life-threatening agranulocytosis.

2. Antipsychotic drugs bind to dopamine receptors and block the action of _____.

3. The major clinical indication for use of antipsychotic drugs is_____.

4. _____ is a drug used to treat psychosis and is metabolized in the liver and excreted in urine and bile.

5. _____ is approved only for the treatment of Tourette's syndrome.

6. The prototype of "atypical" agents is _____.

7. _____ is an antipsychotic drug that is used only for its antiemetic, sedative, and antihistaminic effects.

8. _____ is indicated only when other antipsychotic drugs are ineffective because of its association with cardiac dysrhythmias.

9. _____ _____ are more likely to occur with the older antipsychotic drugs than with the newer "atypical" agents.

10. _____ is considered a hypersensitivity reaction associated with phenothiazines.

■ Clinical Challenge

Your client is a 58-year-old male who has a long-term history of schizophrenia. He has had frequent readmissions to the psychiatric unit. What assessment data do you need to obtain? Based on the frequent readmissions to the hospital, what would you discuss with your client?

■ Review Questions

1. Your client is a newly diagnosed schizophrenic. Which of the following drugs will his physician most likely prescribe for him?
   a. pimozide (Orap)
   b. risperidone (Risperdal)
   c. sotalol (Betapace)
   d. thioridazine hydrochloride (Mellaril)

2. Which of the following clients would be more likely to experience tardive dyskinesia?
   a. a 32-year-old African American male
   b. a 24-year-old Asian female who has taken haloperidol (Haldol) for 2 weeks
   c. an 18-year-old Caucasian male who has just started loxapine (Loxitane) therapy
   d. a 50-year-old Hispanic female who has taken ziprasidone (Geodon) for 2 years

3. A 28-year-old male was hospitalized 1 week ago for acute psychotic symptoms. He is taking fluphenazine hydrochloride (Prolixin) 6 mg daily. He will least likely experience:
   a. extrapyramidal reactions
   b. hypotension
   c. hypertension
   d. sedation

4. You are talking to the mother of a 19-year-old boy who is exhibiting hostility and hyperactivity, and is very combative. The physician explained that her son is probably experiencing an acute psychosis and will be started on an antipsychotic drug. She asks you how long his agitated behavior will last. An appropriate response would be:
   a. "It will be several weeks before he calms down."
   b. "He will always appear agitated."
   c. "I'm not sure. It's really hard to tell."
   d. "Your son should become less agitated a few hours after the drug therapy is started."

5. Your client has been taking an antacid for 2 months. Her physician prescribes loxapine (Loxitane) for acute psychosis. You understand that the dosage of Loxitane may more than likely be:
   a. 10 mg tid PO
   b. decreased because she is taking an antacid
   c. 250 mg/day because of the antacid
   d. increased because of the interaction with the antacid

6. You have just given your client 5 mg of haloperidol (Haldol) IM. You tell him he should lie down for at least 30 minutes. This will help:
   a. prevent orthostatic hypotension
   b. prevent tissue irritation
   c. increase distribution of the drug
   d. prevent delay of the medication reaching the neurotransmitters

7. Phenothiazines cause all of the following effects in the body except:

   a. central nervous system depression

   b. hypersensitivity reactions

   c. increase in blood pressure

   d. decrease in body temperature

8. Your client is a newly diagnosed schizophrenic and has been started on risperidone (Risperdal). Which of the following could contribute to non-compliance with his drug therapy?

   a. multiple daily doses of risperidone

   b. high cost of his medication

   c. unpleasant odor of the medication

   d. nausea that occurs after each dose of the medication

9. Your client is on chlorpromazine (Thorazine). For the last 2 days, his blood pressure has been 100/70. He has complained of dizziness and weakness, and has not wanted to get out of bed. Which of the following would be an appropriate nursing diagnosis for him?

   a. impaired physical mobility related to sedation

   b. risk of injury related to excessive sedation

   c. altered tissue perfusion related to hypotension

   d. self-care deficit related to psychosis

10. Which of the following side effects would you look for in a client who is taking ziprasidone (Geodon)?

    a. constipation

    b. hypertension

    c. agitation

    d. diarrhea

CHAPTER 10

Drugs for Mood Disorders: Antidepressants and Mood Stabilizers

■ Exercises

Answer the following.

1. Define monoamine neurotransmitter dysfunction associated with depression.

2. Discuss neuroendocrine factors in relation to depression.

3. List three other factors that may contribute to depression.

4. List the three types of antidepressant drugs.

5. Explain the mechanism of action for antidepressant drugs.

6. List foods that contain tyramine, which should be avoided when taking a monoamine oxidase inhibitor (MAOI).

7. List factors considered in antidepressant drug selection.

8. Why are selective serotonin reuptake inhibitors (SSRIs) considered first-choice drugs?

9. Why should clients be given only a 5- to 7-day supply of antidepressants?

10. Describe a tricyclic antidepressant (TCA) overdose.

Fill in the blank.

1. Toxicity occurs with serum lithium levels above _____ mEq/L.

2. _____ is used to help stop smoking.

3. _____ is considered the most common mental illness.

4. Phenothiazines increase the effects of lithium and may increase the risk of _____.

5. _____ can be caused by the serotonin syndrome.

6. Antidepressant effects are due to changes in _____, rather than changes in neurotransmitters.

7. _____ are considered third-line drugs.

8. _____ is the prototype of SSRIs.

9. _____ is not metabolized by the body and is entirely excreted by the kidneys.

10. ____ ____ ____ is a self-prescribed herb that is used for depression.

List adverse effects under each antidepressant group.

TCAs	SSRIs	MAOIs

Match the drug trade name to the generic name.

1. ____ citalopram

2. ____ bupropion

3. ____ amitriptyline

4. ____ isocarboxazid

5. ____ imipramine

6. ____ trazodone

7. ____ paroxetine

8. ____ sertraline

9. ____ nefazodone

10. ____ fluoxetine

a. Tofranil

b. Marplan

c. Prozac

d. Paxil

e. Elavil

f. Celexa

g. Serzone

h. Desyrel

i. Zoloft

j. Wellbutrin

■ Clinical Challenge

Your client is unable to concentrate as you talk with him concerning his treatment plan. He interrupts you numerous times as you try to talk with him about his new medication. He is constantly getting up from his chair and walking around the room. He jumps from one topic to another as you continue to talk with him. He tells you that he knows as much as the doctor does about his problems and that you are taking care of the next president of the United States. From your observations, you suspect that your client has which type of mood disorder? He will more than likely be placed on which drug? How long will it take for his medication to decrease his exhibiting behavior?

▪ Review Questions

1. Your client comes to the clinic complaining of a metallic taste in his mouth, blurred vision, tinnitus, and hand tremors. You question him about taking which of the following drugs?

   a. propranolol (Inderal)

   b. furosemide (Lasix)

   c. lithium carbonate (Eskalith)

   d. sertraline (Zoloft)

2. You are aware that your client has been depressed and is on medication. She has tachycardia and increased respirations, and she is sweating. You conclude that she is experiencing:

   a. a lithium overdose

   b. a TCA overdose

   c. an MAOI overdose

   d. an SSRI overdose

3. The lithium dose has been lowered for your client. You tell him he should have serum levels checked every:

   a. month

   b. 6 weeks

   c. 3 months

   d. 6 months

4. Your client has been taking citalopram (Celexa). She is complaining of dizziness, nausea, and a headache. Before talking with her, you suspect that she has:

   a. increased her dosage to 40 mg daily

   b. either omitted doses or stopped taking the drug

   c. had a drug–drug interaction

   d. been smoking

5. Your client is taking isocarboxazid (Marplan). You caution her about eating:

   a. eggs

   b. aged cheeses

   c. onions

   d. strawberries

6. Your client is being treated for a mood disorder. He is taking nefazodone (Serzone). You stress the importance of reporting to the physician which of the following?

   a. headache

   b. dizziness

   c. dark urine

   d. fatigue

7. Which of the following anticonvulsants is used in mood disorders?

   a. diazepam (Valium)

   b. phenytoin (Dilantin)

   c. lorazepam (Ativan)

   d. carbamazepine (Tegretol)

8. When a client appears depressed, the nurse should assess:

   a. suicidal thoughts

   b. blood pressure

   c. social skills

   d. habits

9. Your client comes to the clinic explaining that her husband wants her to stop taking fluoxetine (Prozac). Before you question her, you suspect that she is experiencing which adverse effect:

   a. headache

   b. dizziness

   c. sexual dysfunction

   d. heavy sedation

10. You are taking care of a 70-year-old woman who is depressed and is on an SSRI. Which of the following will you monitor over the next 3 months?

    a. smoking

    b. weight loss

    c. visual disturbances

    d. blood glucose levels

CHAPTER 11

Antiseizure Drugs

■ Exercises

Match the drug trade name to the generic name.

1. ____ levetiracetam
2. ____ clorazepate
3. ____ zonisamide
4. ____ valproic acid
5. ____ lorazepam
6. ____ phenytoin
7. ____ diazepam
8. ____ carbamazepine
9. ____ oxcarbazepine
10. ____ lamotrigine

a. Valium
b. Depakene (capsules)
c. Lamictal
d. Trileptal
e. Dilantin
f. Tegretol
g. Keppra
h. Ativan
i. Zonegran
j. Tranxene

Fill in the blank.

1. When more than one seizure occurs in a similar pattern, the disorder is called _____.

2. _____ is a common cause of seizures during late infancy and childhood.

3. _____ seizures start in a specific area of the brain.

4. _____ seizures are bilateral and symmetric, and have no defined point of origin.

5. The _____ phase of a seizure is characterized by rapid rhythmic and symmetric jerking movements of the body.

6. The _____ phase of a seizure is characterized by prolonged skeletal muscle contraction.

7. _____ seizures are defined as abrupt alterations in consciousness that last a few seconds.

8. _____ _____ is a life-threatening occurrence associated with tonic-clonic convulsions.

9. The most common adverse effects of phenytoin (Dilantin) affect the _____ and _____ _____.

10. _____ is the drug of choice for status epilepticus.

11. _____ should not be prescribed for children younger than 16 years of age because of a serious skin rash that may occur.

12. _____ is a newer drug given for partial seizures that inhibits abnormal neuronal firing but does not affect normal neuronal excitability.

13. _____ can be substituted for carbamazepine without tapering the dose.

14. The dosage of _____ should be reduced by one-half for a client with creatinine clearance below 70 mL/min.

15. _____ is used to treat bipolar disorders and to prevent migraine headaches.

16. _____ would not be prescribed for a client who is allergic to sulfonamides.

17. _____ reduces the effects of cardiovascular drugs.

18. Gingival hyperplasia often occurs in clients who take _____.

19. _____ and _____ decrease the effects of oral contraceptives and postmenopausal hormone replacement therapy.

20. _____ is the drug of choice for absence seizures.

■ Clinical Challenge

Your client has had his first seizure since he started taking carbamazepine 2 years ago. He experienced one seizure prior to drug therapy and has been on a dose of 400 mg bid since the seizure. He and his wife are extremely upset. They do not understand why he has had a seizure while on the medication. What assessment data would you obtain in order to respond to their concern?

■ Review Questions

1. In teaching your client the importance of taking her antiseizure drug at the same time each day, you explain that this will:
   a. decrease expected side effects of the drug
   b. help maintain therapeutic blood levels of the drug
   c. prevent further seizures
   d. make it easier for her to remember to take the medication

2. Your client has begun phenytoin therapy. He asks you how long it will take for the drug to work. An appropriate response would be:
   a. "Approximately 7 to 10 days after phenytoin is started, therapeutic blood levels should occur."
   b. "After a maximum of 3 weeks, benefits will be evident."
   c. "There is really no way to know how long it will take the drug to work."
   d. "There should be a decrease in seizure activity."

3. Gabapentin is prescribed for your client. In your discussion about this drug with her, you would explain that:
   a. she should stop taking the drug if she experiences dizziness
   b. she should take the medication on an empty stomach
   c. hypertension will occur
   d. if she has to take an antacid, she should wait at least 2 hours after the gabapentin dose

4. The most common adverse effect of phenobarbital is:
   a. diarrhea
   b. bradycardia
   c. drowsiness
   d. headaches

5. In assessing your client who is to start zonisamide for generalized seizures, you should question him concerning:
   a. episodes of dizziness
   b. his diet
   c. a history of kidney stones
   d. chronic fatigue

6. In children 6 years and under, oral antiseizure drugs are rapidly absorbed and have short half-lives. This explains why:
   a. the rate of metabolism in children is decreased
   b. therapeutic blood levels are reached earlier in children than in adults
   c. children need lower doses of antiseizure drugs per kg of body weight than do adults
   d. excessive sedation is not a concern

7. A client is taking oxcarbazepine. Which of the following lab tests should have been done before drug therapy was started?

   a. cholesterol

   b. partial thromboplastin time (PTT)

   c. creatinine clearance

   d. follicle stimulating hormone (FSH)

8. The most important goal for a client experiencing seizures is to:

   a. take medication as prescribed

   b. experience control over seizures

   c. avoid serious adverse drug effects

   d. keep follow-up appointments with health care provider

9. All of the following are true concerning simple antiseizure drug therapy in relation to combination drug therapy *except*:

   a. decreased compliance by the client

   b. fewer drug–drug interactions

   c. lower costs

   d. fewer adverse effects

10. Your assessment reveals that your client does not take his antiseizure medication as it is prescribed. He stated that not only did the medication make him "sleepy all the time," but it was also expensive. An appropriate nursing diagnosis would be:

    a. ineffective coping related to denial of seizure disorder

    b. deficient knowledge: drug effects

    c. noncompliance: inappropriate use of medication

    d. risk for injury: dizziness related to drug therapy

CHAPTER 12

Antiparkinson Drugs

■ Exercises

Match the following.

1. ____ dopamine

2. ____ levodopa/carbidopa (Sinemet)

3. ____ levodopa (Larodopa, Dopar)

4. ____ amantadine (Symmetrel)

5. ____ selegiline (Eldepryl)

6. ____ carbidopa (Lodosyn)

7. ____ tolcapone (Tasmar)

8. ____ entacopone (Comtan)

a. Antiviral agent used to increase dopamine levels

b. Increases dopamine in the brain by inhibiting its metabolism by monoamine oxidase (MAO)

c. Antiparkinson drug used to decrease the peripheral breakdown of levodopa

d. Ninety percent excreted through the biliary tract

e. Immediate release form of levodopa/carbidopa combination

f. Antiparkinson drug that is contraindicated in clients with liver disease

g. Most effective drug in treating Parkinson's disease

h. Neurotransmitter

Place T (true) or F (false) in each blank.

1. ____ Parkinson's disease occurs in both men and women between 50 and 80 years of age.

2. ____ People with Parkinson's disease have an increase in dopamine and a decrease in acetylcholine.

3. ____ Several drug combinations may be used before the start of levodopa therapy.

4. ____ Clients with Parkinson's disease may become depressed, isolated, and withdrawn.

5. ____ Iron increases absorption of levodopa.

6. ____ When dopaminergic drugs are discontinued, the dosage should be tapered over 1 week.

7. ____ The optimal dose of an antiparkinson drug is the largest one that allows the client to function.

8. ____ A dopamine agonist is given with levodopa/carbidopa to help relieve symptoms of Parkinson's disease.

9. ____ Levodopa becomes more effective after 5 to 7 years of use.

10. ____ Central activity anticholinergic drugs given for Parkinson's disease may cause confusion, agitation, and hallucinations.

Answer the following.

1. What causes Parkinson's disease?

2. Discuss the goal of antiparkinson drug therapy.

3. List two advantages of antiparkinson combination therapy.

4. What effect do antihistamines have on a client who is taking an anticholinergic drug for Parkinson's disease?

5. List side effects of levodopa.

▪ Clinical Challenge

Your client asks you why she has developed dyskinesia. You are aware that she has been taking levodopa for several years. What would your response be? When she asks how long she will experience the involuntary movements of her tongue and mouth, what will you tell her?

▪ Review Questions

1. Your client has been diagnosed with Parkinson's disease but is unable to take levodopa. Which of the following drugs may be used in her treatment plan?

   a. antipsychotic drugs
   b. anticholinergic drugs
   c. antiadrenergic drugs
   d. antiemetic drugs

2. When assessing a client who will probably be placed on levodopa, which of the following would the nurse be concerned about?

   a. narrow-angle glaucoma
   b. urinary retention
   c. dilated pupils
   d. hallucinations

3. To prevent or reduce nausea and vomiting, the nurse would encourage the client to take Sinemet:

   a. without regard to meals
   b. at bedtime
   c. during or right after a meal
   d. 2 hours prior to the noon meal

4. Your client is taking amantadine. Which of the following would be an appropriate nursing diagnosis?

   a. risk for injury: hypotension related to adverse effects of amantadine
   b. risk for injury: ataxia and dizziness related to adverse effects of antiparkinson drug
   c. alteration in nutrition: vomiting related to adverse effects of amantadine
   d. alteration in nutrition: anorexia related to adverse effects of an anticholinergic drug

5. You are working in a neuro clinic and see clients who have Parkinson's disease. When you observe clients who exhibit restlessness, agitation, and confusion, you suspect that:

   a. most are on levodopa/carbidopa combination drug therapy
   b. they are on levodopa therapy
   c. they are not taking the prescribed drugs
   d. they need to be reevaluated for drug therapy

6. Which of the following statements would indicate that the client understands levodopa therapy?

   a. "I will have to cut liver out of my diet."
   b. "If I don't feel better in 2 weeks, I will discontinue the levodopa."
   c. "I will take my medication at night."
   d. "I take an over-the-counter drug when I get a sinus infection."

7. Which instructions should the nurse give an older client who is taking trihexyphenidyl?

   a. "You must adhere to a strict low-sodium diet."

   b. "Avoid extreme heat. Stay inside as much as possible during the summer."

   c. "Adverse effects will be greatly reduced if taken at night."

   d. "Diarrhea is a likely adverse effect."

8. Therapeutic effects of dopaminergic agents usually occur within:

   a. 24 hours

   b. 2 to 3 days

   c. 10 to 14 days

   d. 2 to 3 weeks

9. Your client is taking levodopa/carbidopa. Which of the following adverse effects will you observe for?

   a. hypertension

   b. constipation

   c. cardiac dysrhythmias

   d. blurred vision

10. You are teaching your client about his new drug, trihexyphenidyl. You will stress that he should avoid which of the following?

   a. antihistamines

   b. alcohol

   c. antiemetics

   d. antipsychotics

CHAPTER 13

Skeletal Muscle Relaxants

■ Exercises

Answer the following.

1. Describe conditions that skeletal muscle relaxants are used to treat.

2. Discuss contraindications for the use of skeletal muscle relaxants.

3. What is the goal of treatment when skeletal muscle relaxants are used?

4. List common side effects of cyclobenzaprine (Flexeril).

5. Formulate two nursing diagnoses related to skeletal muscle relaxants.

Fill in the blank.

1. _____ is the only skeletal muscle relaxant that is not central acting.

2. _____ can cause physical dependence if used long term.

3. _____ is used to treat spasticity in spinal cord injuries and multiple sclerosis.

4. _____ is contraindicated in clients with recent myocardial infarctions.

5. _____ is contraindicated in clients with anemias.

6. _____ can be used to treat tetanus.

7. _____ is contraindicated in clients with prostatic hypertrophy.

8. _____ should not be used longer than 3 weeks.

9. _____ and _____ can cause liver damage.

10. _____ may potentially cause fatal hepatitis.

11. Abrupt withdrawal from _____ may cause hallucinations.

12. Parenteral _____ should not be mixed with other drugs in a syringe.

13. When administering IV _____, have the client lie down for at least 15 minutes after administration.

14. _____ can cause hepatotoxicity.

15. Baclofen, dantrolene, and _____ are used in chronic spastic disorders.

■ Clinical Challenge

Formulate three nursing diagnoses related to the use of dantrolene (Dantrium).

■ Review Questions

1. Your client is a 15-year-old male who has cerebral palsy. Which of the following skeletal muscle relaxants would he take for spasticity?
   a. orphenadrine (Norflex)
   b. methocarbamol (Robaxin)
   c. tizanidine (Zanaflex)
   d. metaxalone (Skelaxin)

2. Which of the statements by your client indicates that he has an understanding of baclofen (Lioresal) therapy?
   a. "I will not take the drug if I develop a rash."
   b. "It takes at least 3 hours to feel the effects of my medication."
   c. "That drug is giving me diarrhea."
   d. "I would rather get my medication in an injection than take it by mouth."

3. Your client is experiencing muscle spasms from a four-wheeler accident. He is receiving 10 mg of cyclobenzaprine (Flexeril) tid. Your teaching plan should include which of the following instructions?
   a. Do not take the medication with food.
   b. Do not drive or operate heavy machinery for the first week.
   c. Increase the dosage if needed.
   d. Stop the drug if dizziness occurs.

4. A client is scheduled for surgery in the morning for a herniated spinal disk. He has been experiencing severe muscle spasms for the last 2 weeks. He will more that likely take which of the following skeletal muscle relaxants?
   a. metaxalone (Skelaxin)
   b. baclofen (Lioresal)
   c. dantrolene (Dantrium)
   d. tizanidine (Zanaflex)

5. Which of the following adverse effects may be significant for a client taking tizanidine (Zanaflex)?
   a. drowsiness
   b. dry mouth
   c. hypotension
   d. constipation

6. Which of the following clients would have the highest risk for hepatotoxicity from taking dantrolene (Dantrium) for 2 months?
   a. a 71-year-old female who is taking a cardiac glycoside and a diuretic
   b. a 53-year-old female who is on hormone replacement therapy
   c. a 22-year-old male who is taking a monoamine oxidase inhibitor
   d. a 56-year-old male who is receiving an antihypertensive agent

7. Which of the following is an adverse effect of cyclobenzaprine (Flexeril)?
   a. dry mouth
   b. bradycardia
   c. agitation
   d. insomnia

8. Your client has muscle spasms associated with multiple sclerosis. She is taking baclofen (Lioresal). At times, she needs help with activities. Her 10-year-old daughter has been helping her dress and comb her hair. However, your main concern is her drug therapy. An appropriate goal for the client would be:
   a. experience improved motor function
   b. take medication as prescribed
   c. experience relief from pain
   d. increase self-care in daily living activities

9. When a skeletal muscle relaxant is given for acute muscle spasms, which of the following would indicate a therapeutic effect?

    a. increased tenderness

    b. increased mobility

    c. decreased mobility

    d. decreased ability to maintain posture and balance

10. Your client is receiving dantrolene (Dantrium) 30 mg daily PO. Which of the following should be monitored periodically?

    a. prothrombin time and partial thromboplastin time

    b. urine specific gravity

    c. aspartate aminotransferase and alanine aminotransferase

    d. follicle stimulating hormone (FSH) levels

CHAPTER 14

Anesthetics

■ Exercises

Define the following terms.

1. general anesthesia

2. balanced anesthesia

3. regional anesthesia

4. topical anesthesia

5. peripheral nerve anesthesia

Place T (true) or F (false) in each blank.

1. ____ Serious adverse effects from general anesthesia will normally occur during or within a few hours of major surgery.

2. ____ Gentamicin will decrease the effects of neuromuscular blocking agents.

3. ____ Seizure activity may follow administration of regional anesthesia.

4. ____ Effects of adjunctive drugs given for preanesthetic medication are usually evident within 20 to 30 minutes after the drugs are given.

5. ____ Prilocaine (Citanest) is a topical anesthetic.

6. ____ Field block anesthesia involves injecting an anesthetic agent into the cerebrospinal fluid.

7. ____ Epidural anesthesia is used most often for obstetrical clients in labor and delivery.

8. ____ Artificial ventilation is necessary when using neuromuscular blocking agents.

9. ____ Neostigmine (Prostigmin) is used as an antidote for tubocurarine.

10. ____ The major advantage of general anesthesia is that it causes less central nervous system (CNS) and respiratory depression.

Match the following.

1. ____ propofol (Diprivan)

2. ____ sevoflurane (Ultane)

3. ____ nitrous oxide

4. ____ tubocurarine

5. ____ thiopental sodium (Pentothal)

6. ____ articaine (Septocaine)

7. ____ halothane (Fluothane)

8. ____ lidocaine (Xylocaine)

9. ____ succinylcholine (Anectine)

10. ____ epinephrine

a. Causes bronchodilation

b. Useful in neurosurgery

c. Prototype of nondepolarizing neuromuscular blocking agents

d. Can be added to local anesthetic solutions to pro-long anesthetic effects

e. Does not potentiate cardiac dysrhythmias

f. Used in children who need emergency intubation

g. One of the oldest and safest anesthetics

h. Single dose causes unconsciousness

i. Used for dental and periodontal procedures

j. One of the most widely used local anesthetic drugs

■ Clinical Challenge

You are caring for a 38-year-old female who was in a motor vehicle accident and who is in the intensive care unit. Your client is on a respirator and is receiving atracurium (Tracrium). Why is your client receiving this drug? If your client is given the drug for an extended period, what complications will you look for? How will the development of drug complications interfere with the client's progress to recovery?

■ Review Questions

1. To help prevent your client from having a headache after receiving spinal anesthesia, you encourage her to:

   a. not eat or drink anything for 10 hours

   b. lie flat without a pillow for 8 to 12 hours

   c. walk in the halls every 30 minutes for 4 hours

   d. lie on her right side for 2 hours

2. The nurse anesthetist assigned to your client consults the physician about the medication to use for the client during surgery. Because your client has a history of cardiac dysrhythmias, the physician will not suggest:

   a. Innovar

   b. Forane

   c. Diprivan

   d. Pentothal

3. Your client is to have surgery in 1 week. You question him about his use of ginseng because it can increase the risk of:

   a. hypertension

   b. stroke

   c. bleeding

   d. myocardial infarction

4. You are taking care of a 7-year-old female who is 6 hours postoperative. Compared with adults, she is more likely to develop which of the following complications?

   a. hemorrhage

   b. laryngospasms

   c. cardiac dysrhythmias

   d. hyperthyroidism

5. Anticholinergic drugs are given during surgery to prevent:

   a. muscle relaxation

   b. antiadrenergic effects

   c. hypertension

   d. vagal effects

6. Your client is receiving lidocaine viscous for a sore on his gum caused by his dentures. You should instruct him to:

   a. follow the application with a full glass of liquid

   b. lie down for 30 minutes after application

   c. refrain from eating or drinking for about an hour after application

   d. have someone take his blood pressure prior to the application

7. Your 10-year-old client has a history of asthma. Why would halothane be a good choice for his surgery?

   a. It causes bronchodilation and does not irritate the respiratory mucosa.

   b. It dilates blood vessels in the brain and increases intracranial pressure.

   c. It is less likely to cause ventricular dysrhythmias.

   d. It can depress respirations and produce hypoxemia.

8. Which of the following clients would be at an increased risk for adverse effects of midazolam (Versed)?

   a. a 22-year-old male with a seizure disorder

   b. a 52-year-old female who is postmenopausal

   c. a 65-year-old male with emphysema

   d. a 40-year-old female who has breast cancer

9. Which of the following regional anesthetics is used during labor and delivery?

   a. chloroprocaine (Nesacaine)

   b. prilocaine (Citanest)

   c. procaine (Novocain)

   d. bupivacaine (Marcaine)

10. Your client is to receive ketamine (Ketalar) for a diagnostic procedure. When explaining to her what to expect before, during, and after the procedure, you will inform her that:

    a. she could possibly experience unpleasant dreams or hallucinations

    b. she will be fully awake immediately after the procedure

    c. she may experience a dry mouth several days after the procedure

    d. she will not experience a "hangover" effect from the anesthesia

CHAPTER 15

Substance Abuse Disorders

■ Exercises

Define the following terms.

1. substance abuse

2. drug dependence

3. psychological dependence

4. physical dependence

5. tolerance

List withdrawal signs and symptoms of the following drugs or drug classifications.

1. barbiturates

2. alcohol

3. opiates

4. cocaine

5. nicotine

Place T (true) or F (false) in each blank.

1. ____ Nurses can prevent abuse by promoting the use of nondrug measures when indicated.

2. ____ Volatile solvents are most often abused by men over the age of 40.

3. ____ Phencyclidine (PCP) produces intoxication similar to that of alcohol.

4. ____ It is difficult to predict the effects of marijuana.

5. ____ Mental alertness is associated with nicotine dependence.

6. ____ A person who abuses one drug will probably abuse others.

7. ____ Nicotine is the most abused drug in the world.

8. ____ Alcohol enhances the effects of hypoglycemia.

9. ____ Benzodiazepine agents are the drugs of choice for treating alcohol withdrawal syndrome.

10. ____ There is no antidote for barbiturate overdose.

Match the following.

1. ____ naloxone (Narcan)

2. ____ acetone

3. ____ mescaline

4. ____ amphetamines

5. ____ flumazenil (Romazicon)

6. ____ heroin

7. ____ LSD

8. ____ "crack"

9. ____ dronabinol (Marinol)

10. ____ MDMA (3, 4 methylenedioxymeth-amphetamine)

a. Antidote for benzodiazepines
b. Referred to as "ecstasy"
c. Hallucinogen derived from lysergic acid
d. A legal cannabis preparation
e. A very potent, widely used form of cocaine
f. A volatile solvent
g. Used for narcolepsy
h. A semisynthetic derivative of morphine
i. Hallucinogen that is an alkaloid of the peyote cactus
j. Antidote for opioids

■ Clinical Challenge

You are on staff at a detoxification center. You are caring for a client who is experiencing barbiturate withdrawal. List signs and symptoms you will look for during the first 72 hours. What will the treatment of acute signs and symptoms involve? How long will your client need to be monitored for potential serious complications?

■ Review Questions

1. A client is admitted to the emergency room with multiple, non–life-threatening lacerations from a motor vehicle accident. You are aware that the accident was caused by alcohol ingestion. In obtaining a health history from a family member, you learn that he is on an anticoagulant. Which of the following should you observe for?

   a. decreased urinary output
   b. hypertension
   c. increased bleeding
   d. irritability

2. You work in a detoxification unit in a large hospital. You are assigned to work with clients experiencing alcohol withdrawal. Which of the following drugs would you use in the treatment of your clients?

   a. benzodiazepines
   b. monoamine oxidase inhibitors
   c. cardiac glycosides
   d. tetracyclines

3. Your client is receiving disulfiram (Antabuse) and complains of fatigue, headache, and dizziness. You explain that:
   a. you will ask the doctor to decrease the dose
   b. after about 2 weeks of treatment, the adverse effects usually subside
   c. some people experience less pleasant adverse effects than he has
   d. the adverse effects will continue as long as he is taking the medication

4. Which of the following drugs would you administer to reduce symptoms of hyperactivity associated with alcohol withdrawal?
   a. lansoprazole (Prevacid)
   b. clonidine (Catapres)
   c. metyrose (Demser)
   d. triamcinolone (Aristocort)

5. Abuse of benzodiazepines can cause which of the following?
   a. seizures
   b. insomnia
   c. nightmares
   d. poor motor coordination

6. You are caring for a client who has abused alprazolam (Xanax) for 5 years. She wants to stop taking the drug. Which of the following will you include when discussing withdrawal from this drug?
   a. Withdrawal symptoms usually begin 12 to 24 hours after the last dose.
   b. There will be no noticeable adverse effects.
   c. She may experience a seizure.
   d. She will be given methadone to help decrease withdrawal symptoms.

7. A client who has overdosed on a barbiturate is brought into the emergency room. The family reports that she has been unresponsive for 5 hours. After an artificial airway has been inserted, the nurse would:
   a. begin gastric lavage
   b. start IV fluids
   c. lower body temperature
   d. administer an emetic

8. You are caring for a client who abuses cocaine. Which of the following vital signs would you expect to find when assessing him?
   a. BP 98/50; P 120; R 40
   b. BP 130/88; P 92; R 28
   c. BP 150/90; P 80; R 16
   d. BP 170/98; P110; R 20

9. Even though marijuana is illegal and not used for therapeutic purposes in the United States, it is useful in treating nausea and vomiting associated with anticancer drugs and in decreasing:
   a. intraocular pressure
   b. hypotension
   c. urinary output
   d. blood glucose levels

10. Assessment of an emergency room client reveals an elevated blood pressure, heart rate, and temperature; dilated pupils; and delusional thought processes. These symptoms indicate ingestion of:
    a. an opiate
    b. an amphetamine
    c. a hallucinogen
    d. a cannabinoid

CHAPTER 16

Central Nervous System Stimulants

■ Exercises

Fill in the blank.

1. _____ is a sleep disorder associated with "sleep attacks" during the day.

2. _____ increase norepinephrine, dopamine, and possibly serotonin in the brain.

3. Carbamazepine (Tegretol) can decrease the effects of _____.

4. _____ is the most common drug used in children for attention deficit-hyperactivity disorder (ADHD).

5. _____ given for narcolepsy may increase the effects of phenytoin (Dilantin).

6. _____ and sodium benzoate are sometimes used as a respiratory stimulant in neonates.

7. _____ is an over-the-counter drug used by college students to keep them from sleeping.

8. _____ is occasionally used as a respiratory stimulant.

9. _____ is contraindicated with a history of ventricular hypertrophy.

10. Central nervous system (CNS) stimulation is an adverse effect of _____.

List the following beverages according to the greatest amount of caffeine to the least amount of caffeine.

1. Iced tea

2. Espresso

3. Coke

4. Diet Pepsi

5. Mountain Dew

6. Mr. Pibb

7. Instant tea

Place a check in the appropriate box if the drug is used in narcolepsy and/or ADHD.

Drug	Narcolepsy	ADHD
Amphetamine		
Dexedrine		
Provigil		
Adderall		
Desoxyn		
Focalin		
Ritalin		

■ Clinical Challenge

Your client is a trial attorney who has narcolepsy. What potential problems do you see for him? Which drug might be prescribed to enable him to continue his profession? What is the expected outcome of drug therapy related to narcolepsy?

■ Review Questions

1. Your adult client is taking methylphenidate (Ritalin) for narcolepsy. He is to receive 40 mg bid. Which of the following times would be best for him to take his medication?

   a. 6 AM and 4 PM

   b. 8 AM and 8 PM

   c. 10 AM and 6 PM

   d. 10 PM and 6 AM

2. All of the following are considered desirable outcomes for clients who are taking CNS stimulants prescribed for narcolepsy except:

   a. balancing the checkbook

   b. raking leaves in the yard

   c. operating the lawnmower

   d. napping every day

3. In teaching a client who ingests several soft drinks a day to decrease caffeine intake, your instructions would be to avoid:

   a. Coke

   b. Mountain Dew

   c. Pepsi

   d. Dr. Pepper

4. Which of the following clients could safely use a CNS stimulant?

   a. a 38-year-old Caucasian female with glaucoma

   b. a 65-year-old African American male who experiences angina

   c. a 50-year-old male who has adult-onset diabetes

   d. a 28-year-old African American female with hyperthyroidism

5. A 6-year-old is taking methamphetamine (Desoxyn), 10 mg daily for ADHD. At each clinic visit, the nurse should assess:

   a. height and weight

   b. vision

   c. temperature

   d. blood pressure

6. A mother of a young client being treated for ADHD is concerned about her child having to take medication. An appropriate response to her would be:

   a. "The medication is needed to help your son function in society."

   b. "Without the medication, your son would not be able to go to school."

   c. "We can discuss the adverse effects of his medication if you like."

   d. "Hopefully, the medication can be omitted during the summer when he is out of school."

7. A client is being instructed on the use of modafinil (Provigil) for narcolepsy. Which of the following best reflects an expected goal of client-teaching activities related to the drug?

   a. Client will be able to identify two adverse effects of the drug.

   b. Family members will understand why the client must take the drug.

   c. Client will understand the physiological action of modafinil.

   d. Client will exercise three times a week.

8. Which of the following activities would the nurse be responsible for during the evaluation phase of drug therapy for a child receiving methylphenidate (Ritalin) for ADHD?

   a. preparation and administration of the drug

   b. ongoing monitoring of the child for therapeutic effects

   c. establishing outcome criteria related to the drug therapy

   d. gathering data related to a drug history

9. Counseling a mother concerning her 4-year-old daughter's treatment of ADHD would include the importance of:

    a. well-balanced meals

    b. increased physical activities

    c. limiting social encounters

    d. using sunscreen when outside

10. Which drug increases the effects of modafinil (Provigil)?

    a. furosemide (Lasix)

    b. glipizide (Glucotrol)

    c. carbamazepine (Tegretol)

    d. buspirone (Buspar)

CHAPTER 17

Physiology of the Autonomic Nervous System

■ Exercises

Match the following.

1. ____ homeostasis

2. ____ desensitization

3. ____ ligands

4. ____ muscarinic receptors

5. ____ somatic nervous system

6. ____ norepinephrine

7. ____ nicotinic receptors

8. ____ hypersensitization

9. ____ acetylcholine

10. ____ autonomic nervous system

a. Controls voluntary activities in the visceral organs of the body

b. Increase in beta-adrenergic responsiveness

c. Located in most internal organs

d. Innervates skeletal muscle and controls voluntary movement

e. A main neurotransmitter of the autonomic nervous system

f. Located in motor nerves and skeletal muscle

g. Neurotransmitters, hormones, or medications that bind to receptors

h. Synthesized from amino acid tyrosine

i. Decrease in beta-adrenergic responsiveness

j. Constant internal environment

Fill in the blank.

1. _____ neurons carry sensory input from the periphery to the central nervous system.

2. Decreased heart rate is the body's response to _____ stimulation.

3. _____ receptors allow calcium ions to move into the cell and produce muscle contraction.

4. The _____ nervous system includes all the neurons and ganglia found outside the central nervous system.

5. _____ impulses travel from the central nervous system along the preganglionic nerves to ganglia.

6. _____ acts on alpha and beta receptors.

7. _____ neurons transport motor signals from the central nervous system to the peripheral areas of the body.

8. _____ are comprised of the terminal end of the preganglionic nerve and clusters of postganglionic cell bodies.

9. Increased muscle strength is the body's response to _____ stimulation.

10. _____ acts mainly on alpha receptors.

■ Review Questions

1. Which term is used to describe a drug that has the same effects on the body as stimulation of the peripheral nervous system?
   a. adrenergic
   b. cholinergic
   c. sympathomimetic
   d. parasympatholytic

2. The physiological action of nicotine receptors is to:
   a. inhibit respiratory response
   b. excite the cardiovascular system
   c. produce muscle contraction
   d. increase intracellular concentration of calcium

3. Adrenergic fibers secrete:
   a. epinephrine
   b. norepinephrine
   c. acetylcholine
   d. dopamine

4. Which adrenergic neurotransmitter is necessary for normal brain function?
   a. acetylcholine
   b. catecholamine
   c. dopamine
   d. epinephrine

5. Beta$_1$ adrenergic receptors are found in the:
   a. blood vessels
   b. liver
   c. kidney
   d. heart

6. A specific body response to parasympathetic stimulation is:
   a. dilated pupils
   b. increased motility of the gastrointestinal tract
   c. increased heart rate
   d. decreased secretions from sweat glands

7. Parasympathetic nervous system responses are regulated by:
   a. dopamine
   b. cyclic adenosine monophosphate (cAMP)
   c. norepinephrine
   d. acetylcholine

8. A specific body response to the "fight-or-flight" reaction is:
   a. increased muscle strength
   b. decrease in breakdown of muscle glycogen
   c. decrease in sweating
   d. increase in secretions from the lungs

9. The automatic nervous system is regulated by centers in the central nervous system, including the:
   a. thyroid gland
   b. pituitary gland
   c. hypothalamus
   d. adrenal medullae

10. A function of alpha$_1$ adrenergic receptors is:
    a. relaxation of intestinal smooth muscle
    b. increased heart rate
    c. bronchodilation
    d. aggregation of platelets

CHAPTER 18

Adrenergic Drugs

■ Exercises

List five commonly used adrenergic drugs in each category.

Alpha and beta activity	Alpha activity	Beta activity

Match the following drugs with indications for their clinical use. Some may be used more than once; some may not be used at all.

1. ____ Tuamine
2. ____ Aramine
3. ____ Levophed
4. ____ Privine
5. ____ Ephedrine
6. ____ Neo-Synephrine
7. ____ Intropin
8. ____ Adrenalin
9. ____ Afrin
10. ____ Visine

a. Vasoconstriction in the eye
b. Gout
c. Cardiac stimulation
d. Hyperglycemia
e. Nasal decongestion
f. Ophthalmic conditions
g. Hypotension and shock
h. Hypertension
i. Diuresis
j. Bronchodilation

Place T (true) or F (false) in each blank.

1. ____ Topical decongestants can be used for 10 days.

2. ____ Many over-the-counter preparations contain adrenergic drugs.

3. ____ Adrenergic drugs are given to decrease blood pressure.

4. ____ Antihistamines may increase the effects of adrenergic drugs.

5. ____ Acute bronchospasm is most often relieved within 5 minutes of administration of epinephrine.

6. ____ You should not aspirate when giving epinephrine in a tuberculin syringe.

7. ____ The use of an adrenergic drug in a critically ill client may result in hyperglycemia.

8. ____ Liver disease is a contraindication to use of adrenergic drugs.

9. ____ The most common use of epinephrine in children is for the treatment of asthma.

10. ____ Pseudoephedrine toxicity occurs with doses four to five times greater than the normal dose.

■ Clinical Challenge

Your client is to be given epinephrine for laryngeal edema associated with anaphylactic shock. How much epinephrine will you administer and in what type of syringe? What can the nurse do to accelerate relief of symptoms? How long should it take for the client to experience some relief?

■ Review Questions

1. When discussing nasal decongestants with a client in the allergy clinic, the nurse will impart information regarding:
   a. rebound congestion
   b. foods to be avoided
   c. compliance with allergy injections
   d. environmental factors

2. Your client is to have surgery and will have a general anesthetic. You will question her concerning the use of adrenergic drugs because of increased risk of:
   a. bronchial relaxation
   b. mydriasis
   c. cardiac dysrhythmias
   d. emotional disturbances

3. Which of the following drugs would be contraindicated for use with adrenergic drugs because of a potentially fatal outcome?
   a. Dopram
   b. Marplan
   c. Elavil
   d. Ritalin

4. You have administered tetrahydrozoline hydrochloride (Visine) 1 gtt OU. An expected outcome would be:
   a. decreased redness
   b. pupil constriction
   c. decreased tear activity
   d. improved accommodation

5. Which route of administration is not used for epinephrine?
   a. inhalation
   b. injection
   c. oral
   d. topical

6. The client is experiencing a serious allergic reaction to a bee sting. Epinephrine is administered to relieve:
   a. pain and swelling around the sting site
   b. itching of skin around the site
   c. anxiety
   d. acute bronchospasm and laryngeal edema

7. A client has been taking pseudoephedrine (Sudafed) for sinuses. Which of the following adverse effects may he experience?
   a. bradycardia
   b. hypertension
   c. hypoglycemia
   d. hypothyroidism

8. Your client is a diabetic and is on insulin therapy. During treatment of acute asthmatic bronchitis, the nurse should assess:
   a. partial thromboplastin time level
   b. blood glucose level
   c. blood pressure
   d. urinary output

9. When teaching a client about the use of tetrahydrozoline hydrochloride (Visine), the nurse should advise which of the following?

    a. Wear a hat when outdoors.

    b. Drink a liter of fluid each day.

    c. Do not wear soft contact lenses while using the drug.

    d. Rest the eyes at least once every 2 to 3 hours.

10. The nurse has administered isoproterenol to a client who is in shock. An expected outcome would be which of the following?

    a. decreased pulse

    b. decreased blood pressure

    c. increased blood pressure

    d. increase in body temperature

CHAPTER 19

Antiadrenergic Drugs

■ Exercises

Answer the following.

1. Why are alpha$_1$ blocking agents used in benign prostatic hyperplasia (BPH)?

2. List five effects on the body caused by beta-adrenergic blocking agents.

3. What is the goal of antiadrenergic drug therapy?

4. Describe the blocking effects of antiadrenergic drugs.

5. What is the physiological action of alpha$_2$ agonist drugs?

Indicate the clinical use for each beta-adrenergic blocking agent by placing a check in the appropriate column.

Drug	Angina	Myocardial infarction	Dysrhythmias	Hypertension	Glaucoma	Migraine
Atenolol						
Metoprolol						
Nadolol						
Propanolol						
Acebutolol						
Esmolol						
Sotalol						
Timolol						
Betaxolol						
Carteolol						
Levobunolol						
Metipranolol						

■ Clinical Challenge

A client is admitted to the hospital complaining of chest pains, palpitations, and shortness of breath. Blood pressure is 138/86, pulse is 94, and respirations are 24. After an extensive cardiac evaluation, she is sent home on propranolol (Inderal). Why was propranolol (Inderal) prescribed for this client? What information should the nurse tell the client about this drug? How long will the client take the drug?

■ Review Questions

1. The home health nurse is caring for a diabetic client who is taking metipranolol (OptiPranolol) for glaucoma. She will observe for:
   a. weight gain
   b. hypoglycemia
   c. headaches
   d. hyperglycemia

2. Clients who have received beta blockers after a myocardial infarction should be monitored for:
   a. hypertension and respiratory distress
   b. hypotension and heart failure
   c. hypertension and hyperthyroidism
   d. hyponatremia and kidney failure

3. Your client has cirrhosis and is taking tamsulosin (Flomax) for BPH. The nurse anticipates that the client will receive:
   a. a lower than usual dose of the drug
   b. twice as much as the usual dose
   c. a combination dose
   d. a normal adult dose

4. Early administration of a beta blocker after an acute myocardial infarction can decrease the occurrence of:
   a. renal failure
   b. heart block

   c. ventricular dysrrhythmias
   d. respiratory depression

5. Which of the following beta blockers is most frequently used in children?
   a. propranolol (Inderal)
   b. sotalol (Betapace)
   c. pindolol (Visken)
   d. nadolol (Corgard)

6. Your client is starting methyldopa (Aldomet) for hypertension. You would instruct the client to take the medication:
   a. on an empty stomach
   b. first thing in the morning
   c. with food
   d. at bedtime

7. An expected outcome for a client with benign prostatic hyperplasia who is on an alpha-blocking agent would be:
   a. increased blood pressure
   b. improved urination
   c. decreased blood glucose
   d. decreased sex drive

8. An adverse effect of propranolol that should be discussed with a client is:
   a. dizziness with activity
   b. excessive sleeping
   c. increased anxiety in crowds
   d. rapid weight loss

9. Your client is taking Aldomet. You would question her concerning her use of:
   a. steroids
   b. vitamins
   c. oral contraceptives
   d. sedatives

10. A client is leaving the hospital on a beta blocker. He has had a history of angina in the past but there are no major cardiac concerns at this time. Which of the following should he report to his physician?
    a. a weight gain of more than 2 pounds a week
    b. excessive energy
    c. a decreased appetite
    d. insomnia

■Diagram

Fill in the blanks in Figure 19-1 with the terms below.

Myocardial or other tissue cells
Beta-adrenergic blocking drugs
Epinephrine and norepinephrine
Nerve endings
Receptor site

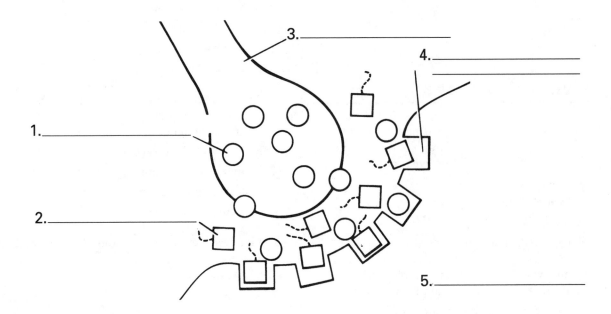

FIGURE 19-1.

CHAPTER 20

Cholinergic Drugs

■ Exercises

Fill in the blank.

1. Cholinergic drugs stimulate the _____ nervous system.

2. In myasthenia gravis, autoantibodies destroy _____ receptors for acetylcholine, which causes muscle weakness to occur.

3. The only therapeutic use for an irreversible anticholinesterase inhibitor is in the treatment of _____.

4. _____ is used to treat urinary retention due to urinary bladder atony.

5. _____, _____, and _____ are anticholinesterase agents approved for the treatment of Alzheimer's disease.

6. _____ is the prototype anticholinesterase agent.

7. _____ is used to differentiate between myasthenic and cholinergic crises.

8. _____ _____ is the only anticholinesterase that can cross the blood-brain barrier.

9. _____ is the maintenance drug of choice for clients with myasthenia gravis.

10. _____ can delay progression of Alzheimer's disease up to 55 weeks.

11. _____ is a drug used in the treatment of Alzheimer's disease that is metabolized by the liver and excreted in feces.

12. _____ is a centrally acting anticholinesterase agent that can cause hepatotoxicity.

13. _____ can be used in the neonate of a mother who has myasthenia gravis.

14. _____ can be used in severe cases of anticholinergic poisoning as an antidote.

15. _____ is a specific antidote to cholinergic agents.

Place T (true) or F (false) in each blank.

1. ____ Ingestion of clitocybe mushrooms causes cholinergic crises.

2. ____ All people who have myasthenia gravis require a caregiver to administer their medication.

3. ____ Myasthenia gravis is an autoimmune disorder.

4. ____ Cholinergic stimulation results in decreased peristalsis.

5. ____ Acetylcholine stimulates cholinergic receptors to promote normal urination.

6. ____ Direct-acting cholinergic drugs decrease respiratory secretions.

7. ____ Cholinergic drugs are contraindicated in peptic ulcer disease.

8. ____ Cholinergic drugs produce miosis.

9. ____ The best route for administration of bethanechol (Urecholine) is the oral route.

10. ____ Because of its duration of action, rivastigmine (Exelon) can be taken twice a day.

▪ Clinical Challenge

A 52-year-old female has been diagnosed with myasthenia gravis. Her treatment plan includes pyridostigmine (Mestinon). Why would it be important to encourage the client or a family member to record symptoms associated with myasthenia gravis in relation to the effects of the drug therapy?

▪ Review Questions

1. Your client has a confirmed diagnosis of myasthenia gravis and is started on pyridostigmine (Mestinon). The nurse is aware of the following adverse effect of pyridostigmine:

   a. dry mouth

   b. nausea

   c. constipation

   d. urinary retention

2. A 73-year-old man has been diagnosed with Alzheimer's disease and is started on tacrine (Cognex). Client instruction would include:

   a. Renal function should be monitored for 3 months.

   b. Cardiac enzymes should be monitored indefinitely.

   c. White blood cell count should be checked every month.

   d. Liver function should be monitored for at least 6 months.

3. It would be important to tell a client who has started on neostigmine (Prostigmin) that:

   a. he should limit fluids for a few days

   b. the drug could cause constipation

   c. he will take an oral form of the drug once a day for 5 days

   d. the drug acts within 1 hour of administration

4. The client, age 69, has a diagnosis of myasthenia gravis. She is experiencing abdominal cramping, diarrhea, weakness, and difficulty breathing. The nurse suspects cholinergic crisis and prepares which of the following?

   a. atropine 0.6 mg IV

   b. atropine 1.0 mg IM

   c. atropine 0.4 mg subq

   d. atropine 0.5 mg PO

5. A client's daughter calls the clinic and states that her mother, age 73, appears to be extremely dizzy. After questioning the daughter, you determine that the mother has Alzheimer's disease and is taking donepezil (Aricept). The nurse will be most concerned about the possibility of:

   a. headaches during the morning

   b. orthostatic hypotension

   c. injury while ambulating

   d. nausea and vomiting

6. You are working in a women's hospital where you are caring for a new mother who is experiencing postpartum urinary retention. Bethanechol (Urecholine) has been ordered. To prevent nausea and vomiting, you will administer the medication:

   a. before meals

   b. during meals

   c. after meals

   d. with a full glass of milk

7. Which of the following drugs decrease the effects of cholinergic agents?

   a. corticosteroids

   b. aminoglycoside antibiotics

   c. antihyperglycemics

   d. antihistamines

8. Your client has myasthenia gravis and is receiving pyridostigmine (Mestinon). She is complaining of nausea and vomiting. An appropriate response to her would be:

   a. "I'm so sorry, but that is to be expected."

   b. "Try taking your medication with food."

   c. "I'll talk to your doctor about decreasing the dose."

   d. "Make sure you get plenty fluids during the day."

9. Parenteral bethanechol (Urecholine) is administered by which route:

a. oral

b. subcutaneous

c. intramuscular

d. intravenous

10. When neostigmine (Prostigmin) is given for postoperative distention, which of the following would indicate increased gastrointestinal muscle tone and motility?

a. absence of flatus through the rectum

b. increased urination

c. presence of bowel sounds

d. absence of bowel movements

CHAPTER 21

Anticholinergic Drugs

■ Exercises

Match the following.

1. ____ ipratropium (Atrovent)

2. ____ trihexyphenidyl (Trihexy)

3. ____ benztropine (Cogentin)

4. ____ atropine

5. ____ flavoxate (Urispas)

6. ____ oxybutynin (Ditropan)

7. ____ tolterodine (Detrol)

8. ____ belladonna tincture

9. ____ scopolamine

10. ____ homatropine hydrobromide (Homapin)

a. Used in the treatment of parkinsonism and extrapyramidal reactions

b. Most often used for antispasmodic effects

c. Antimuscarinic, anticholinergic agent used to treat urinary frequency and urgency

d. Useful in treating rhinorrhea due to allergy or common cold

e. Increases bladder capacity

f. Useful in treating cystitis

g. Used to treat acute dystonic reactions

h. Prototype anticholinergic drug

i. Used for motion sickness

j. Ocular effects do not last as long as with atropine

Answer the following.

1. Describe the mechanism of action for anticholinergic drugs.

2. List five specific effects of anticholinergic drugs on the body.

3. Why are anticholinergic drugs given prior to surgery?

4. Why is atropine given with meperidine (Demerol) to relieve severe pain with renal colic?

5. List signs and symptoms of anticholinergic overdose.

6. How do tertiary amines and quaternary amines differ?

7. Why are oral anticholinergic drugs not given to treat asthma?

8. Why is the use of cyclopentolate (Cyclogyl) and tropicamide (Mydriacyl) guarded in children?

9. List five adverse effects associated with the use of anticholinergic drugs in the elderly.

10. Why do large doses of anticholinergic drugs cause facial flushing?

■ Clinical Challenge

Formulate three nursing diagnoses and a client goal for each in relation to anticholinergic drug therapy.

■ Review Questions

1. A client is being discharged from the hospital and will be taking dicyclomine (Bentyl) for irritable bowel syndrome. It will be important to instruct the client to:

   a. take the medication on an empty stomach

   b. limit intake of red meat

   c. take the drug 30 minutes before meals and at bedtime

   d. avoid drinking caffeinated beverages

2. You are a nurse in a large eye clinic and work in the client education department. You are working with a client who is receiving homatropine (Homapin). It is important to teach her:

   a. to stop the medication and call her physician if eye pain occurs

   b. that she cannot wear her contacts

   c. that she should rest her eyes two to three times a day

   d. that her visual acuity will decrease with use of the drug

3. Which of the following drugs can increase the effects of anticholinergic drugs?

   a. cardiac glycosides

   b. antihistamines

   c. anti-inflammatory agents

   d. oral hypoglycemics

4. Your client is 68 years old and is planning a cruise to Mexico. In anticipation of "sea sickness," he asks you for medication to prevent this. You suggest that his physician may prescribe a scopolamine patch but caution him concerning:

   a. heat stroke

   b. urinary retention

   c. decreased saliva

   d. diarrhea

5. Because of their adverse effect, urinary retention, anticholinergic drugs should not be prescribed for clients with:

   a. chronic constipation

   b. increased blood pressure

   c. prostatic hypertrophy

   d. urinary tract infections

6. Your client is planning a deep-sea fishing trip. He will take Transderm-V to protect him against motion sickness. You instruct him that a dose will provide protection for:

   a. 12 hours

   b. 24 hours

   c. 36 hours

   d. 72 hours

7. A client is receiving oxbutynin (Ditropan) for a neurogenic bladder. An expected outcome of this drug is:

    a. decreased frequency of voiding

    b. increased frequency of voiding

    c. decreased bladder capacity

    d. increased urgency in voiding

8. A client has been taking glycopyrrolate (Robinul) for adjunctive management of peptic ulcer disease for 3 years. The nurse questions him concerning:

    a. chronic diarrhea

    b. dental hygiene practices

    c. headaches

    d. diet

9. Anticholinergic drugs are contraindicated in which of the following?

    a. diabetes mellitus

    b. rheumatoid arthritis

    c. hyperthyroidism

    d. bradycardia

10. Your client has been taking propantheline bromide (Pro-Banthine) for irritable bowel syndrome. She tells you that the medication is making her constipated and confused at times. She states that she has missed a few doses because the "pills just cost too much." An appropriate nursing diagnosis for your client would be:

    a. constipation related to decrease in gastrointestinal motility

    b. disturbed thought process: confusion

    c. impaired urinary elimination: decreased bladder tone and urine retention

    d. noncompliance related to adverse drug effects and cost of the medication

CHAPTER 22

Physiology of the Endocrine System

■ Exercises

Place T (true) or F (false) in each blank.

1. _____ Hormones initiate cellular reactions and functions.

2. _____ Steroid hormones are water-soluble and can easily cross cell membranes.

3. _____ Most hormones from endocrine glands are secreted into the bloodstream and act on distant organs.

4. _____ A peptide is a protein-derived hormone.

5. _____ Water-soluble hormones have a long duration of action.

6. _____ Some hormones may act as a "first messenger" to cells.

7. _____ Cyclic adenosine monophosphate (cAMP) is considered a first messenger for some hormones.

8. _____ Malfunction of an endocrine organ is most often associated with hyposecretion or inappropriate secretion of its hormones.

9. _____ Drugs are more often given for endocrine gland hypofunction than for hyperfunction.

10. _____ Malfunction of endocrine organs can cause death.

Fill in the blank.

1. Hormones act as _____ _____ to transmit information within the body.

2. _____ is a hormone that is produced by the kidneys and stimulates bone marrow to produce red blood cells.

3. White blood cells produce _____ that act as messengers among leukocytes in the inflammatory process.

4. The _____ connects the nervous system and the endocrine system.

5. _____, _____, and _____ _____ are secreted in 24-hour cycles.

Answer the following.

1. List the major organs of the endocrine system.

2. List the body activities that are regulated by the endocrine system.

3. Give an example of how one hormone can affect different body tissues.

4. Describe two mechanisms that eliminate hormones from the body.

▪ Review Questions

1. The hormone that stimulates bone marrow to produce red blood cells is:

   a. secretin

   b. glucagon

   c. cholecystokinin

   d. erythropoietin

2. Which of the following best describes hormones given for physiologic effects?

   a. small doses of hormones given as a replacement or substitute for the amount of hormone normally secreted

   b. the same amount of hormone given that would normally be secreted

   c. hormones given that have more potent and prolonged effects than naturally occurring hormones

   d. large doses of hormones given for greater effects than the amount normally secreted

3. The connection between the nervous system and the endocrine system is the:

   a. thyroid gland

   b. hypothalamus

   c. pancreas

   d. pituitary gland

4. An example of a hormone that affects specific target tissue is:

   a. prolactin

   b. peptides

   c. corticotropin

   d. secretin

5. Which of the following is not an effect of ovarian estrogen?

   a. promotion of ovarian follicle maturation

   b. stimulation of the endometrial lining of the uterus to promote its growth and cyclic changes

   c. promotion of uterine contractions during labor

   d. stimulation of breast tissue to promote growth of milk ducts

6. Which of the following statements best describes water-soluble, protein-derived hormones?

   a. have a longer duration of action because they are bound to plasma proteins

   b. have a short duration of action and are inactivated by enzymes in the liver and kidneys

   c. are conjugated in the liver to inactive forms and excreted in bile or urine

   d. are inactivated by enzymes at receptor sites on target cells

7. Calmodulin is an intracellular regulatory protein that activates protein kinases when bound to:

   a. calcium

   b. phospholipids

   c. cAMP

   d. adenyl cyclase

8. Which of the following hormones is secreted in a 24-hour cycle?

   a. epinephrine

   b. growth hormone

   c. progestin

   d. estrogen

9. Receptors in target organs for hormones may be increased or decreased in response to:

   a. hormone binding to receptors

   b. changes in the secretions produced by cells

   c. malfunction of the endocrine organ involved

   d. chronic exposure to abnormal levels of hormones

10. Hypofunction of an endocrine gland can result from:

    a. inappropriate response of intracellular metabolic processes

    b. excessive stimulation of the gland

    c. enlargement of the gland

    d. a hormone-producing tumor

CHAPTER 23

Hypothalamic and Pituitary Hormones

■ Exercises

Match the following.

1. ____ corticotropin-releasing hormone

2. ____ hypophyseal stalk

3. ____ anterior pituitary

4. ____ serotonin

5. ____ thyrotropin-releasing hormone

6. ____ somatotropin

7. ____ follicle-stimulating hormone

8. ____ antidiuretic hormone

9. ____ posterior pituitary

10. ____ Cushing's disease

a. Stores and releases hormones synthesized in the hypothalamus

b. Neurotransmitters that stimulate the secretion of corticotropin-releasing hormones

c. Anatomically connects the hypothalamus and pituitary gland

d. Used in diagnostic tests of pituitary function and hyperthyroidism

e. Stimulates functions of sex glands

f. Stimulates growth of body tissues

g. Released in response to stress or threatening stimuli

h. A disorder characterized by excessive cortisol

i. Regulates water balance in the body

j. Composed of glandular cells that synthesize and secrete hormones

Place T (true) or F (false) in each blank.

1. ____ Corticotropin-releasing hormone is secreted during the night.

2. ____ There are many uses for hypothalamic and pituitary hormones.

3. ____ Vasopressin enables corticotropin-releasing hormone to stimulate adrenocorticotropic hormone (ACTH) secretion.

4. ____ Most all hormones are administered or taken orally.

5. ____ Somatostatin inhibits the release of the growth hormone.

6. ____ Norepinephrine stimulates secretion of corticotropin-releasing hormone.

7. ____ Hypothalamic hormones are rarely used in most clinical settings.

8. ____ The growth hormone-releasing hormone is found only in the hypothalamus.

9. ____ Elevated levels of glucocorticoids decrease or prevent the ability of corticotropin-releasing hormone to stimulate ACTH secretion.

10. ____ Pituitary hormones are given to replace or supplement naturally occurring hormones.

Provide the name of each hormone beside its abbreviation.

1. TRH _____

2. GnRH _____

3. FSH _____

4. LH _____

5. PIF _____

6. ACTH _____

7. TSH _____

8. CRH _____

9. ADH _____

10. CRF _____

■ Clinical Challenge

A client, age 55, develops diabetes insipidus following surgery for removal of a pituitary tumor. He is started on vasopressin (Pitressin) 0.25 mL SQ bid. Why has the client been placed on vasopressin? What adverse effects may the client experience? What will the nurse include in the discharge teaching?

■ Review Questions

1. Your client, age 7, has a deficiency of endogenous growth hormone. She is started on somatropin (Humatrope) 0.03 mg/kg IM three times a week. Before the physician administers the first injection, you will check documentation for which of the following?

   a. evidence of open bone epiphyses

   b. daily urine output

   c. daily fluid input

   d. understanding of drug therapy

2. In teaching parents about growth hormone therapy for their child, the nurse will be sure to include:

   a. reporting the type of exercise the child participates in weekly

   b. monitoring the child's height and weight regularly

   c. recording the food intake daily

   d. administering the medication weekly

3. A mother whose child is taking growth hormone therapy reports that her child is complaining of localized muscle pain. The nurse's response should be:

   a. "Adverse effects are very common."

   b. "The muscle pain will go away. Don't worry about it."

   c. "You may give her Tylenol. If she still experiences pain, let me know."

   d. " You will need to limit her physical activity."

4. Your client, age 9, has been taking somatrem (Protropin) for 3 years. On routine clinic visits, the nurse will monitor:

   a. blood pressure

   b. urine protein levels

   c. heart rate

   d. blood glucose levels

5. Your client has diabetes insipidus and is receiving desmopressin (DDAVP). During your 9 PM rounds, you notice that he is confused and lethargic. Upon questioning him, you determine that he has a headache and is nauseated. You suspect he is experiencing:

   a. water intoxication

   b. depression

   c. dehydration

   d. an allergic reaction

6. You are working in the postpartum unit. Three of your clients are receiving oxytocin (Pitocin) to control postpartum bleeding. In observing for therapeutic effects in each client, you will expect to find:

   a. decreased vaginal bleeding and a firm uterine fundus

   b. intense uterine contraction and decreased vaginal bleeding

   c. a soft, round uterus and moderate vaginal bleeding

   d. cessation of vaginal bleeding and a large, soft uterine fundus

7. Which of the following is a common adverse effect of octreotide (Sandostatin)?

   a. nausea

   b. symptoms of gallstones

   c. hypoglycemia

   d. constipation

8. Your client is diagnosed with diabetes insipidus and is placed on vasopressin (Pitressin). You will expect to administer this drug by which of the following routes?

   a. oral

   b. intradermal

   c. intramuscular

   d. intravenous

9. Which of the following would indicate that vasopressin is producing its therapeutic effect in your client?

   a. increased signs of dehydration

   b. decreased urine output

   c. decreased urine specific gravity

   d. increased thirst

10. When assessing a client who is taking vasopressin (Pitressin), the nurse will report which of the following?

    a. increased temperature

    b. decreased blood pressure

    c. thirst

    d. sore throat

CHAPTER 24

Corticosteroids

■ Exercises

Fill in the blank.

1. Corticosteroids are contraindicated in systemic _____ infections.

2. Cortisol, corticosterone, and cortisone are examples of _____.

3. _____ is the main mineralocorticoid.

4. _____ is the prototype of corticosteroid drugs.

5. _____ is given to clients with liver disease.

6. The absence of _____ in the body causes death.

7. _____ decrease the effects of corticosteroids.

8. _____ _____ is used to treat Crohn's disease.

9. Adrenal _____ are responsible for few of the physiologic effects of the sex hormones.

10. In treating chronic asthma, _____ corticosteroids are drugs of first choice.

Place T (true) or F (false) in each blank.

1. ____ Excessive corticosteroid secretion damages body tissues.

2. ____ Corticosteroids are secreted directly into the bloodstream.

3. ____ High plasma levels of cortisol cause excessive corticotropin secretion.

4. ____ Only a few adrenal corticosteroids are available as drug preparations.

5. ____ Hydrocortisone and cortisone are most often the drugs of choice for adrenocortical insufficiency.

6. ____ Corticosteroid therapy for children is calculated according to weight.

7. ____ During periods of stress, corticosteroid therapy must be increased.

8. ____ Corticosteroids are given locally rather than systemically to prevent systemic toxicity.

9. ____ Parenteral administration of corticosteroids is indicated for all clients.

10. ____ The body's normal response to critical illness is decreased secretion of cortisol.

Answer the following.

1. Explain the process that has to occur before corticosteroids are secreted.

2. Why is the use of corticosteroids in children a major concern?

3. Discuss how dietary changes can be helpful in reducing some adverse effects of corticosteroid therapy.

4. Give one example of a corticosteroid whose duration of action lasts 48 hours.

5. Why is prednisone often the drug of choice for anti-inflammatory, antiallergic, antistress, and immunosuppressive disorders treated by a corticosteroid with primarily glucocorticoid activity?

▪ Clinical Challenge

Your client has been diagnosed with primary adrenocortical insufficiency (Addison's disease) due to cancer. Outline your teaching plan related to replacement therapy. How will the diagnosis of cancer affect your plan?

▪ Review Questions

1. Your client is an 81-year-old male who has been on long-term prednisone therapy for rheumatoid arthritis. During your assessment of him, which of the following signs might you find related to chronic steroid use?

   a. poor vision
   b. thin, easily injured skin
   c. dry, flaky skin
   d. decreased hearing

2. Which of the following would be the most appropriate nursing diagnosis for a client taking steroids?

   a. imbalanced nutrition: less than body requirements
   b. deficient fluid volume
   c. risk for infection
   d. ineffective breathing pattern

3. Your client has been on an oral corticosteroid for 3 weeks. He tells you that he has missed several doses. An appropriate response to him would be:

   a. "Don't worry about it. It will not affect the intended outcome."
   b. "Alteration in administration of the drug can cause complications."
   c. "Next time you miss a dose, take an extra tablet with the next dose."
   d. "You really should be more careful in taking your medication."

4. Your client has a diagnosis of adrenocortical insufficiency and is steroid dependent. She has just lost her husband in a motor vehicle accident. During this time of stress, her medication will be:

   a. the same
   b. decreased
   c. increased
   d. discontinued

5. Your client is taking flunisolide (Nasalide) for allergic rhinitis. On her most recent visit to the allergy clinic, she tells you she has gained 20 pounds. You assess for:

   a. increased activity
   b. potassium intake
   c. sodium intake
   d. use of alcohol

6. The nurse will encourage the client to take which of the following medications at a different time rather than with the prescribed corticosteroid?

   a. Ampicillin

   b. Mylanta

   c. Advil

   d. Dramamine

7. Your client has Addison's disease and is taking cortisone (Cortone) 50 mg daily PO. An expected outcome of cortisone therapy for your client would be:

   a. increased energy level

   b. weight gain

   c. increase in blood pressure

   d. constipation

8. Your client, age 53, has severe asthma. She has taken prednisone (Deltasone) for years. Recently, her physician has started her on alternate-day therapy. She tells you she would rather take her medication every day. Which of the following would be your best response?

   a. "This schedule will be more convenient for you."

   b. "This schedule will enable you to lose weight."

   c. "This schedule will decrease the cost of your medication."

   d. "This schedule allows rest periods so that adverse effects are decreased but the anti-inflammatory effects continue."

9. Your client is taking fludrocortisone (Florinef) 0.1 mg daily PO for chronic adrenocortical insufficiency. Client teaching for him will always include:

   a. taking his medication on an empty stomach

   b. promoting a diet high in potassium

   c. discouraging activity

   d. stopping the medication if drowsiness occurs

10. Your client is admitted to the emergency room in acute respiratory distress related to severe asthma. Which of the following conditions should the nurse assess for prior to administering methylprednisolone sodium succinate (Solu-Medrol)?

    a. peptic ulcer disease

    b. urinary retention

    c. irritable bowel syndrome

    d. sinus infection

CHAPTER 25

Thyroid and Antithyroid Drugs

■ Exercises

Fill in the blank.

1. Production of thyroxine and triiodothyronine depends on the presence of _____ and _____ in the thyroid gland.

2. _____ _____ is an enlargement of the thyroid gland resulting from iodine deficiency.

3. Synthetic _____ is the drug of choice in treating hypothyroidism.

4. Tyrosine is an amino acid derived from dietary _____.

5. _____ is the drug of choice for long-term treatment of hypothyroidism.

6. _____ drugs inhibit synthesis of thyroid hormones and do not damage the thyroid gland.

7. _____ preparations inhibit the release of thyroid hormones and cause them to be stored within the gland.

8. Levothyroxine is converted to _____ in peripheral tissues.

9. Serum _____ levels are used to monitor thyroid hormone replacement.

10. Thyroid hormones act by controlling _____ _____ _____.

Match the following.

1. ____ Synthroid
2. ____ Euthroid
3. ____ Propylthiouracil
4. ____ Cytomel
5. ____ Tapazole
6. ____ Lugol's solution
7. ____ Iodotope
8. ____ Inderal
9. ____ Methimazole
10. ____ saturated solution of potassium iodide

a. Prototype of the thioamide antithyroid drugs

b. Used to treat short-term hyperthyroidism and as an expectorant

c. Used to treat symptoms of hyperthyroidism involving stimulation of the sympathetic nervous system

d. Synthetic preparation of T_3

e. Can be used to treat children with hyperthyroidism

f. Drug of choice for long-term treatment of hypothyroidism

g. Used to treat thyroid cancer

h. Similar to propylthiouracil (PTU), is well absorbed and reaches peak plasma levels quickly

i. Used to treat thyrotoxic crisis

j. Similar to composition of natural thyroid hormone

Place T (true) or F (false) in each blank.

1. ____ Thyroxine is more potent than triiodothyronine.

2. ____ The thyroid gland extracts iodine from the circulating blood.

3. ____ The thyroid-stimulating hormone (TSH) stimulates the thyroid gland to release thyroid hormones into circulation.

4. ____ Thyroid hormones influence very few cells in the body.

5. ____ Hypothyroidism and hyperthyroidism produce opposing effects on the body.

6. ____ To compensate for decreased production of thyroid hormone, the anterior pituitary gland secretes less TSH.

7. ____ Simple goiter is common in the United States.

8. ____ Iodine preparations reduce serum levels of thyroid hormones more quickly than do thioamide drugs.

9. ____ Taking levothyroxine on an empty stomach decreases absorption of the drug.

10. ____ Thyroid replacement therapy in clients with hypothyroidism is lifelong.

▪ Clinical Challenge

Your client, a 42-year-old female, has been diagnosed with hypothyroidism. She is placed on Synthroid 0.05 mg/day PO. She is concerned that her dose may have to be increased. What do you tell her in response to her concern? What will be included in your teaching plan for her?

▪ Review Questions

1. Which of the following is an initial indication that your client has primary hypothyroidism?
   a. serum TSH of 5.2 microunits/L
   b. serum TSH of 0.1 microunits/L
   c. serum TSH of 0.5 microunits/L
   d. serum TSH of 3 microunits/L

2. Your client has been diagnosed with hyperthyroidism. You expect that an appropriate nursing diagnosis related to her weight would be:
   a. imbalanced nutrition: less than body requirements
   b. imbalanced nutrition: more than body requirements
   c. swallowing: impaired
   d. oral mucous membranes: altered

3. An expected outcome for your patient who has been on thyroid medication would be:
   a. decreased pulse rate
   b. increased blood pressure
   c. increased energy and activity levels
   d. decreased appetite

4. Your client has been recently started on levothyroxine (Synthroid). All of the following would be included in the teaching plan *except*:
   a. Never take over-the-counter drugs unless the physician has been consulted.
   b. Avoid the herb ephedra.
   c. Synthroid may be switched to Levothroid.
   d. Limit intake of caffeine beverages to two or three a day.

5. Your client is taking levothyroxine (Levothroid) and explains to you that occasionally he has to take an antacid for heartburn. Your best response to him would be:
   a. "Take the two medications together."
   b. "You should not take an antacid when taking Levothroid."
   c. "Take your thyroid medication 2 hours before you take the antacid."
   d. "Skip the Levothroid dose when you take the antacid."

6. Your client, age 28, has primary hypothyroidism and is taking levothyroxine (Synthroid). She asks you how long she will have to take the medication. Your response to her would be:

   a. "Just for a few weeks."

   b. "You will take the medication for 1 year, then your physician will taper your dose for a few months."

   c. "Usually, people with hypothyroidism will need to take their medication for the rest of their lives."

   d. "Don't worry about that now. We will discuss it later."

7. Your client is 25 years old and is on thyroid hormone replacement. She is also taking an oral contraceptive. You suspect that her thyroid medication will need to be:

   a. increased

   b. decreased

   c. kept the same

   d. discontinued

8. Propranolol (Inderal) is given to your client who has been diagnosed with hyperthyroidism. This drug:

   a. enhances the effects of PTU

   b. controls symptoms resulting from excessive stimulation of the sympathetic nervous system

   c. converts levothyroxine hormone to liothyronine (T_3).

   d. replaces the thyroid hormone from an exogenous source.

9. Your client has been placed on PTU. Your assessment data reveal that he is on medication for high blood pressure and high cholesterol. Due to the change in the rate of body metabolism from the PTU, you expect the physician to:

   a. discontinue the other medications

   b. increase the dosage of blood pressure medication

   c. keep the dosages of the other two medications the same

   d. reduce the dosage of the blood pressure and cholesterol medication

10. Your client is taking PTU for hyperthyroidism. Which of the following instructions should be given to him concerning administration of his medication?

   a. Take the medication every 8 hours around the clock.

   b. Take the medication once daily.

   c. If a dose is missed, double the next dose.

   d. Take the daily dose at bedtime.

CHAPTER 26

Hormones That Regulate Calcium and Bone Metabolism

▪ Exercises

Fill in the blank.

1. Calcium and bone metabolism are regulated by
   _____ _____, _____, and
   _____.

2. _____ is a hormone from the thyroid
   gland whose secretion is regulated by the
   concentration of ionized calcium in the blood
   flowing through the thyroid gland.

3. Clinical manifestations of hyperparathyroidism
   are those of _____.

4. _____ raises serum calcium levels by
   increasing intestinal absorption of calcium and
   mobilizing calcium from the bone.

5. In osteoporosis, _____ prevents further
   bone loss in the presence of adequate calcium
   and vitamin D.

6. _____ is a synthetic preparation used to
   treat Paget's disease that can cause nausea and
   facial flushing.

7. _____ is a selective estrogen receptor
   modulator and is used for prevention of
   postmenopausal osteoporosis.

8. _____ is classified as an anti-estrogen and
   is used to prevent and treat breast cancer.

9. A nonprescription antacid that is used as a
   calcium supplement is _____.

10. _____ inhibits bone mineralization and
    may cause osteomalacia.

Answer the following.

1. List five disorders of calcium and bone disorders.

2. Describe the pharmacokinetics of
   bisphosphonates.

3. How does calcitonin lower serum calcium levels?

4. List five functions of calcium.

5. Why is phosphorus one of the most important
   elements in normal body function?

Fill in the chart.

Category	Calcium requirement
Normal adult	
Growing child	
Pregnant woman	
Lactating woman	
Postmenopausal woman	

▪ Clinical Challenge

Your 65-year-old client has been told by her
physician that she is at risk for osteoporosis. He has
suggested that she begin alendronate (Fosamax). She
asks you why she should take this medication. What
would your response be? Which drugs would you
question your client about that could predispose a

woman to osteoporosis? What instructions would you give your client regarding alendronate (Fosamax)?

■ Review Questions

1. Your client is taking calcitriol (Rocaltrol) and is complaining of headaches, nausea, drowsiness, and muscle weakness. You suspect that she has:
   a. hypocalcemia
   b. hypercalcemia
   c. hypokalemia
   d. hyperkalemia

2. Your client complains that having to sit in an upright position after taking alendronate (Fosamax) is inconvenient. Your explanation to her would include that the upright position:
   a. is necessary for proper absorption of the drug
   b. is not necessary
   c. allows for a faster metabolism and excretion of the drug
   d. helps prevent esophageal irritation and stomach upset

3. A client in the emergency room is being treated for hypercalcemia. The physician orders an injection of calcitonin (Calcimar). You are aware that the serum calcium level should decrease in:
   a. 30 minutes
   b. 1 hour
   c. 2 hours
   d. 3 hours

4. Which of the following should be included when instructing a client on how to take tetracycline and calcium preparations?
   a. Take the drugs at the same time.
   b. Take the drugs 2 to 3 hours apart.
   c. Do not take calcium supplements when taking tetracycline.
   d. Take the tetracycline 30 minutes after taking the calcium supplement.

5. During your initial assessment of a client, you discover that she is taking digoxin and a calcium supplement for hypocalcemia. You should assess for signs of:
   a. anemia
   b. digitalis toxicity
   c. hyponatremia
   d. Paget's disease

6. Which of the following drugs used to treat osteoporosis increases bone formation?
   a. vitamin D
   b. raloxifene (Evista)
   c. teriparatide (Forteo)
   d. alendronate (Fosamax)

7. Your client has renal impairment and is being treated for osteomalacia. Which of the following drugs is she most likely to be taking?
   a. calcitriol (Rocaltrol)
   b. alendronate (Fosamax)
   c. risedronate (Actonel)
   d. zoledronate (Zometa)

8. Your client is to start vitamin D therapy. You learn that he has cirrhosis of the liver. You suspect that he will take:
   a. dihydrotachysterol (Hytakerol)
   b. paricalcitol (Zemplar)
   c. calcitriol (Rocaltrol)
   d. calcifediol (Calderol)

9. Hypocalcemia is the diagnosis for your client. Prior to drug therapy, you would expect his serum calcium level to be:
   a. below 8.5 mg/dL
   b. between 5.2 and 10 mg/dL
   c. above 12 mg/dL
   d. above 20 mg/dL

10. Which of the following would be an expected outcome for a client taking alendronate (Fosamax) for osteoporosis?
    a. decreased bone mass density
    b. presence of Chvostek's sign
    c. absence of bone fractures
    d. decreased serum calcium level

CHAPTER 27

Antidiabetic Drugs

■ Exercises

Match the following.

1. _____ polyuria

2. _____ oral antidiabetic drugs

3. _____ hypoglycemia

4. _____ glycogenolysis

5. _____ insulin

6. _____ polydipsia

7. _____ hyperglycemia

8. _____ ketoacidosis

9. _____ polyphagia

10. _____ glucose

a. Increased appetite

b. Major stimulus of insulin secretion

c. Some of these drugs can lower blood sugar by decreasing absorption or production of glucose

d. Blood glucose below 60 to 70 mg/dL

e. Increased urine output

f. A life-threatening complication that occurs with severe insulin deficiency

g. Breakdown of glycogen

h. A protein hormone secreted by beta cells in the pancreas

i. Characterized by excessive thirst, hunger, and increased urine output

j. Increased thirst

Place T (true) or F (false) in each blank.

1. _____ Insulin is the only drug used to treat type 1 diabetes.

2. _____ Insulin is never given to clients with type 2 diabetes.

3. _____ Insulin is contraindicated in hypoglycemia.

4. _____ Insulin can be given orally.

5. _____ Insulin that has been refrigerated should be used within 1 year.

6. _____ Metformin is often the initial drug of choice in obese clients with newly diagnosed type 2 diabetes.

7. _____ Glitazones are contraindicated in clients with liver disease.

8. _____ Ginseng increases blood glucose levels.

9. _____ Dosage of insulin must be individualized according to blood glucose levels.

10. _____ Insulin can be given with all types of oral antidiabetic drugs.

11. _____ Clients with diabetic ketoacidosis have an increase of insulin in the body.

12. _____ There are higher levels of insulin in clients with hepatic impairment because less insulin is metabolized.

13. _____ Insulin is absorbed faster from the upper arm than the abdomen.

14. _____ Regular insulin and isophane insulin (NPH) require a prescription.

15. _____ Symptoms of hypoglycemia are excess thirst, hunger, and increased urine output.

16. ____ Symptoms of hyperglycemia include sweating, nervousness, weakness, tremors, and mental confusion.

17. ____ One-half of the insulin that is secreted reaches systemic circulation.

18. ____ Epinephrine raises blood glucose levels, which can stimulate insulin secretion.

19. ____ Glucosuria appears when the blood glucose level is four times the normal value.

20. ____ Omitting or decreasing insulin dosage may lead to ketoacidosis.

Fill in the chart, where applicable, for oral hypoglycemic drugs.

Drug	Classification	Onset of action	Peak	Duration	Special considerations
metformin (Glucophage)					
acarbose (Precose)					
glipizide (Glucotrol)					
glimepiride (Amaryl)					
pioglitazone (Actos)					
repaglinide (Prandin)					

Complete the chart for the different types of insulin.

Type	Onset	Peak	Duration
Regular Iletin II			
NPH			
Humalog			
Humulin N			
Lente I			
Ultralente			
Novolin R			

■ Clinical Challenge

1. Your client is a 48-year-old Native American. She has been diagnosed with type 2 diabetes. She is 50 pounds overweight and has known allergies to sulfa drugs. Which oral antidiabetic drug will she most likely be started on? What information will be considered in the selection of her medication?

■ Review Questions

1. You are teaching a mother of a newly diagnosed diabetic child how to assess for hypoglycemia. Which of the following signs will you include?

   a. increased urine output

   b. increased hunger

   c. shakiness/nervousness

   d. excessive thirst

2. Before a client is started on metformin (Glucophage), he should be assessed for which of the following?

   a. renal disease

   b. anemia

   c. osteoporosis

   d. hypertension

3. Your client has been controlled on 30 U of NPH insulin for several years. Recently, he was placed on prednisone for rheumatoid arthritis. You suspect that, due to the prednisone therapy, the NPH dosage may:

   a. stay the same

   b. need to be increased

   c. be discontinued for a short period

   d. need to be decreased

4. A client who takes NPH insulin asks you about the use of an insulin pump. In considering her question, you are aware that which of the following insulins is used in a pump?

   a. NPH

   b. Ultralente

   c. Lente

   d. Regular

5. A 38-year-old client is receiving 30 U of NPH insulin and 8 U of regular insulin at 7:30 AM. She is receiving 25 U of NPH insulin and 5 U of regular insulin at 3:30 PM. Her blood glucose levels have been elevated by 10:30 AM for the last several days. What adjustments should be made in her insulin therapy?

   a. Both morning doses of NPH and regular insulin should be increased.

   b. The morning dose of regular insulin should be increased.

   c. Both afternoon doses should be increased.

   d. The afternoon NPH dose should be increased.

6. A client receives 25 units of NPH insulin at 8 AM. At what time of day should the nurse be alert for a potential hypoglycemic reaction?

   a. after breakfast

   b. before breakfast

   c. at bedtime

   d. before dinner (evening meal)

7. Your client has been on metformin (Glucophage) for 5 years. He is scheduled for major surgery in 2 weeks. You inform him that:

   a. his metformin dose will increase

   b. he will be taken off of metformin and placed on insulin therapy during surgery and for some time after surgery

   c. he will take metformin as prescribed during and after surgery

   d. he will not need to take therapy for diabetes during or after surgery

8. Your client will be taking insulin lispro (Humalog). What instructions do you need to give to him concerning the administration of this drug?

   a. Take 1 hour before meals.

   b. Take at bedtime only.

   c. Take 1½ hours after meals.

   d. Take 15 minutes prior to meals.

9. Your client has just been diagnosed with type 1 diabetes and is placed on regular and NPH insulin. When teaching her about self-administration of her medication, you will most likely advise her to:

   a. administer medications separately in two syringes

   b. administer both medications in one syringe, drawing up the regular insulin first

   c. administer the regular insulin first, then check the blood sugar to determine whether NPH is needed

   d. administer both medications together, drawing up the NPH insulin first

10. Which of the following statements from your client indicates a need for further education regarding diabetes therapy?

    a. "I will need more insulin on the days I take my aerobics class."

    b. "I wear a medical alert bracelet stating that I am diabetic at all times."

    c. "I get a family member to check my syringe and make sure I have drawn up the correct dose of insulin."

    d. "I know that I should eat my meals at regularly scheduled times."

CHAPTER 28

Estrogens, Progestins, and Oral Contraceptives

■ Exercises

Place T (true) or F (false) in each blank.

1. _____ Estrogens and progestins are synthesized from cholesterol.

2. _____ Small amounts of estrogens are found in adipose tissue.

3. _____ Estrone is the major estrogen.

4. _____ During pregnancy, the placenta produces small amounts of estriol.

5. _____ When fertilization does not take place, levels of estrogen and progesterone increase.

6. _____ If an ovum is fertilized, progesterone acts to maintain the pregnancy.

7. _____ Most hormonal contraceptives are synthetic estrogen and progestin.

8. _____ Decreased pituitary stimulation of the ovaries may result in estrogen replacement therapy.

9. _____ Women who take hormones should have a complete physical every 3 years.

10. _____ Oral contraceptives increase the effects of insulin.

Answer the following.

1. Describe the main function of estrogen.

2. Why is progestin used in hormone replacement therapy?

3. List five contraindications to hormone therapy.

4. Describe the three mechanisms of hormonal contraception.

5. Why is estrogen contraindicated in pregnancy?

Fill in the blank.

1. _____ is secreted by the corpus luteum during the last half of the menstrual cycle.

2. Estrogens are inactivated in the _____.

3. During pregnancy, increased levels of _____ cause the uterus and breast to enlarge and relaxation of the ligaments and joints in the pelvis.

4. _____ prepares the breasts for lactation by promoting development of milk-producing cells.

5. The most widely used synthetic steroid estrogen is _____ _____.

6. _____ _____ is an herb used to treat symptoms of menopause.

7. _____ is the only drug approved by the FDA for postcoital contraception.

8. _____ is used as a transdermal patch that releases slowly into the vascular system.

9. _____ is approved for short-term treatment of hot flashes and sweating.

10. _____ are contraindicated in clients with impaired liver function or liver disease.

■ Clinical Challenge

Your client, age 48, comes to the health clinic with symptoms of postmenopausal syndrome. She complains of fatigue, hot flashes, and increased perspirations. What assessment data will you obtain from the client? Your client is placed on hormone replacement therapy. Outline a teaching plan for her.

■ Review Questions

1. A 19-year-old female is seen in the clinic for unprotected sexual intercourse the night before. She is requesting emergency contraception. Which of the following drugs will she be given?
   a. Estraderm
   b. Prempro
   c. Preven
   d. Cenestin

2. Your client has been placed on hormone replacement therapy. Provera has been prescribed for her. She should be instructed that she is at risk for:
   a. colon cancer
   b. gall bladder disease
   c. Alzheimer's disease
   d. osteoporosis

3. A client who has been placed on estrogen complains of nausea. The nurse should instruct her to:
   a. eat six small meals a day
   b. take her medication before breakfast
   c. drink a full glass of water with each pill
   d. take medication after meals or at bedtime

4. Your client will be using estradiol skin patches for hormone replacement therapy. You teach her that she should apply the patch:
   a. to the abdomen
   b. to her breast
   c. in the waistline area
   d. on the forearm

5. Your client has a history of seizures and is taking carbamazepine. Her physician has just prescribed an oral contraceptive for her. The client will be informed that she should:
   a. use an additional birth control method
   b. stop taking her seizure medication
   c. ask her neurologist about decreasing her dose of carbamazepine
   d. take her seizure medication at night with her oral contraceptive

6. A client has been placed on Premarin 1 mg daily. The nurse will advise which of the following in her teaching session with the client:
   a. Take the medication only when needed.
   b. Report to the emergency room if nausea occurs.
   c. Avoid exercise.
   d. Monitor her weight.

7. You are assessing a client who will be placed on hormone replacement therapy. Which of the following data would cause immediate concern?

   a. walking 2 miles a day

   b. cigarette smoking

   c. eating large meals

   d. occasional headaches

8. A client has requested to be placed on hormone replacement therapy for severe hot flashes and fatigue. She has been told that she is not a good candidate for hormone replacement therapy. You suspect she has a history of:

   a. kidney disease

   b. liver disease

   c. asthma

   d. osteoporosis

9. Your client has been taking birth control pills for 3 years. She calls the clinic to tell you that she has had a stomach virus and has been unable to take her pills for 2 days. Which of the following responses would be appropriate?

   a. "Take three pills today and continue as prescribed."

   b. "Take two pills now!"

   c. "You need to speak to your physician."

   d. "Take two pills today and two tomorrow, then continue as prescribed."

10. Which of the following would indicate a contraindication to birth control pills?

    a. frequent headaches

    b. calf tenderness

    c. weight loss

    d. dizziness

CHAPTER 29

Androgens and Anabolic Steroids

■ Exercises

Answer the following.

1. Name three organs of the body that secrete androgens.

2. List the three functions of testosterone.

3. Why are androgens and anabolic steroids classified as Schedule III drugs?

4. List 10 potentially serious side effects of anabolic steroids.

Fill in the blank.

1. Male sex hormones are synthesized from _____.

2. Androgens produced by the ovaries are used as precursor substances for the production of naturally occurring _____.

3. _____ is the only important male sex hormone.

4. _____ is a transdermal form of testosterone that has a rapid onset of action and lasts approximately 24 hours.

5. Testoderm must be applied to the _____ to achieve adequate blood levels.

6. _____ may be used to prevent or treat endometriosis or fibrocystic breast disease in women.

7. _____ inhibits the metabolism of carbamazepine and increases risks of toxicity.

8. Androgens and anabolic steroids are contraindicated in clients with preexisting _____ disease.

9. Testosterone is secreted by _____ cells in the testes in response to stimulation by the luteinizing hormone from the anterior pituitary gland.

10. Testosterone increases protein _____ and decreases protein _____.

■ Clinical Challenge

You and your spouse are at a social gathering. Someone asks you what you think of the rumor going around town about the high school football team and anabolic steroids. What would your response be?

■ Review Questions

1. Your client has acquired primary hypogonadism and is to begin testosterone therapy. Testoderm has been prescribed. He is instructed to apply the patch to his:
   a. forearm
   b. scrotum
   c. buttocks
   d. upper back

2. A client is to start testosterone therapy. Testoderm TTS has been prescribed. The health care provider instructs him to change the patch:
   a. every 12 hours
   b. daily
   c. every 3 days
   d. weekly

3. A 62-year-old is on androgen therapy. The nurse will inform him of which of the following possible adverse effects?
   a. increased sperm count
   b. increased libido
   c. high-pitched voice
   d. increased pubic hair

4. A 13-year-old client takes testosterone because his father had delayed puberty. The client will be assessed for which of the following every 6 months?
   a. migraine headaches
   b. altered long bone growth
   c. hyperglycemia
   d. increased hair growth

5. You work in a women's clinic. You are aware that women who are unresponsive to conventional therapy for endometriosis are given which of the following?
   a. danazol (Danocrine)
   b. testosterone enanthate (Delatestryl)
   c. testosterone cypionate (Depo-Testosterone)
   d. methyltestosterone (Methitest)

6. Your client, age 48, is taking testosterone for hypogonadism due to an androgen deficiency. Which of the following lab tests should be monitored during therapy?
   a. renal blood urea nitrogen (BUN) and creatinine levels
   b. cardiac enzymes
   c. sperm count levels
   d. hepatic function levels

7. Your client, age 15, is taking testosterone. You suspect he is concerned about his appearance. Which of the following nursing diagnoses would be appropriate for him?
   a. disturbed self-esteem
   b. disturbed personal identity
   c. deficient knowledge
   d. ineffective sexuality patterns

8. Your client is prepubescent and has been taking testosterone for cryptorchidism. Follow-up care would include:
   a. monthly creatinine levels
   b. radiograph of hand and wrists every 6 months
   c. weekly blood glucose levels
   d. monthly partial thromboplastin time levels

9. A client, 62 years old, who has been on warfarin (Coumadin) for some time has recently been diagnosed with androgen deficiency and has been placed on testosterone (Testoderm). Which of the following should be monitored?

a. prothrombin time

b. serum creatinine

c. blood glucose level

d. BUN level

10. A 56-year-old female has been placed on testolactone (Teslac) for breast cancer. Which of the following will likely be a concern for her?

a. high blood pressure

b. increase in appetite

c. excessive growth of hair

d. headaches

CHAPTER 30

Nutritional Support Products and Drugs for Obesity

■ Exercises

Match the following.

1. ____ pancreatin (Creon)

2. ____ glucomannan

3. ____ LipoKinetix

4. ____ phentermine (Ionamin)

5. ____ Nepro

6. ____ kilocalories

7. ____ guarana

8. ____ sibutramine (Meridia)

9. ____ guar gum

10. ____ orlistat (Xenical)

a. Most frequently prescribed adrenergic anorexiant

b. Drug used for obesity with controversy concerning deaths

c. A source of commercial caffeine found in weight loss products

d. A combination dietary supplement associated with severe hepatotoxicity

e. Preparation of pancreatic enzymes used to aid in digestion

f. Dietary fiber found in weight-loss products

g. Drug used for obesity that decreases absorption of dietary fat from intestines

h. A high-calorie, low-electrolyte enteral formulation

i. Herb that produces feelings of stomach fullness

j. Measurement of energy

Place T (true) or F (false) in each blank.

1. ____ Appetite suppressants should be taken at night to decrease appetite the next day.

2. ____ An indication of water deficit is drowsiness.

3. ____ When taking orlistat, if a meal is missed, the dose can be omitted.

4. ____ Carbohydrates and fats serve as sources of energy for cellular metabolism.

5. ____ When oral or tube feedings are contraindicated, providing nutritional supplements of intravenous fluids may be used for the short term.

6. ____ Obesity is more likely to occur in men.

7. ____ Fewer children are developing type 2 diabetes due to obesity.

8. ____ The most commonly reported adverse effects of phentermine, an adrenergic anorexiant, are nervousness, dry mouth, constipation, and hypertension.

9. ____ Most preparations for weight loss cause cardiovascular problems.

10. ____ Antacids may increase the effects of pancreatic enzymes.

Complete the chart.

Formula	Nutritional value	Uses
Enfamil		
	Contains less phenylalanine	Infants and children with phenylketonuria
Pregestimil		
Prosobee		Infants who are allergic to milk
Isocal		
	Complete; contains an easily digested form of fat	Clients with fat malabsorption problems
		Clients with severe burns, trauma, or sepsis
	Provides amino acids, carbohydrates, and some electrolytes	Clients with renal failure
Nutrivent		
Polycose	Oral supplement	
	Complete	Children 1–6 years of age

■ Clinical Challenge

1. A 56-year-old female with recurring colon cancer is recovering from extensive surgery involving the colon, one kidney, the bladder, one fallopian tube, and the uterus. She is sent home 10 days postoperatively. After 4 days of being at home, her husband calls her physician and tells him that she cannot eat, has lost 8 pounds, and is lethargic. She is readmitted into the hospital and started on parenteral feedings. Why is the client receiving parenteral feedings? The husband asks how long she will receive the parenteral feeding. What will your response be?

The physician discharges the client, and she is to continue the feedings at home. What will be your instructions?

■ Review Questions

1. Phentermine (Ionamin), an adrenergic anorexiant, has been prescribed for your client. Which of the following conditions is a contraindication to the use of this drug?
   a. diabetes mellitus
   b. cardiovascular disease
   c. chronic fatigue syndrome
   d. confusion

2. Which of the following statements by your client leads you to believe that she has a good understanding of the drug orlistat (Xenical)?
   a. "I hate having to take the medication three times a day."
   b. "I no longer have a lot of gas."
   c. "I take a multivitamin with my morning dose of Xenical."
   d. "I shouldn't have as many bowel movements as I have been having."

3. Your client comes to the clinic complaining about the "bad" taste of MCT oil. She indicates that she is going to stop drinking the preparation. Your response to her should be:
   a. " I'll talk to your doctor and see whether we can change your enteral preparation."
   b. "Mix it with water and drink it as fast as you can."
   c. "You may mix this preparation with your favorite fruit juice."
   d. "I know. It tastes terrible. I would stop taking it, too."

4. You are in charge of orientation for new RN graduates who are working in a long-term care facility. When instructing them concerning intermittent tube feedings, you will advise that:
   a. tubing should be changed every 24 hours
   b. tube placement does not have to checked before feeding
   c. solutions should be heated prior to use
   d. administration should be over a 10-minute period

5. A major complication of tube feeding is:
   a. aspiration of formula into the lungs
   b. irritation of the esophagus
   c. pancreatitis
   d. diarrhea

6. Your client is receiving an intravenous fat emulsion. Which of the following lab values should be checked before administration?
   a. blood glucose levels
   b. serum sodium levels
   c. triglyceride levels
   d. potassium levels

7. Increasing calorie intake for your client who has chronic obstructive pulmonary disease may lead to:
   a. increased carbon dioxide production
   b. decreased carbon dioxide production
   c. decreased need for oxygen
   d. respiratory alkalosis

8. A 78-year-old is admitted to the emergency room with a complaint of excessive vomiting and diarrhea for 6 days. You will note the following signs of water deficit *except*:
   a. increased hematocrit
   b. flushed skin
   c. drowsiness
   d. dry mucous membranes

9. Your client is to begin taking pancrelipase (Viokase). Instructions regarding administration should include taking the medication:
   a. at least 2 hours prior to eating
   b. immediately before or with meals
   c. with a full glass of water
   d. at bedtime

10. You are working with an obese client who tells you that she does not like to leave her house, even to go to the grocery store. She states that she has had her groceries delivered to her home for the past 2 years. Which of the following would be an appropriate nursing diagnosis for her?
    a. chronic low self-esteem related to body image
    b. fluid volume: excess related to excessive intake
    c. imbalanced nutrition, more than body requirements
    d. activity intolerance related to weight

CHAPTER 31

Vitamins

■ Exercises

Match the following.

1. ____ vitamin E

2. ____ vitamin B$_3$ (niacin)

3. ____ vitamin C

4. ____ vitamin K

5. ____ vitamin B$_1$

6. ____ vitamin B$_6$

7. ____ vitamin B$_{12}$

8. ____ vitamin A

9. ____ vitamin B$_2$

10. ____ vitamin D

a. A coenzyme in metabolic processes

b. Functions in production of corticosteroids and red blood cells

c. Essential for energy production

d. Required for normal vision

e. Necessary for collagen formation

f. Functions as an antioxidant

g. Necessary for glycolysis

h. Necessary for normal blood clotting

i. Essential for normal metabolism of all body cells, red blood cells, and growth

j. Important in calcium and bone metabolism

Fill in the blank.

1. Vitamin _____ is given by injection for clients with pernicious anemia.

2. Vitamins _____ and _____ may increase the anticoagulant effect of warfarin (Coumadin).

3. Vitamin _____ may help reduce incidence of lung, breast, and bladder cancers.

4. Vitamin _____ may help reduce incidence of esophagus, stomach, and colon cancers.

5. _____ _____ and vitamin _____ may help prevent cardiovascular disease.

6. _____ is contraindicated in liver disease because it increases liver enzymes and causes further liver damage.

7. Vitamin _____ is found in sweet potatoes, squash, apricots, peaches, and cantaloupe.

8. Vitamin _____ can be found in vegetable oils.

9. Adequate intake of _____ _____ can prevent severe birth defects in infants.

10. _____ causes blood vessels to dilate, causing facial flushing, dizziness, and falls.

Define the following.

1. Dietary reference intake (DRI)

2. Recommended dietary allowance (RDA)

3. Adequate intake (AI)

4. Estimated average requirement (EAR)

5. Tolerable upper intake level (UL)

▪ Clinical Challenge

A male who is thought to be homeless is brought into the emergency room. It is determined that he is an alcoholic. His emaciated condition causes concern for medical conditions. In treating his nutritional state, which vitamins will be ordered for him?

Describe nursing care related to this client. What is the likelihood that this client will comply with a medical regime?

▪ Review Questions

1. You have an 18-year-old client who has a seizure disorder and takes carbamazepine. In preparation for the future, the nurse suggests she take which of the following vitamins to prevent birth defects?

   a. folic acid

   b. retinol

   c. niacin

   d. riboflavin

2. Your client is taking niacin for treatment of hyperlipidemia. Which of the following would be included in client teaching concerning this vitamin?

   a. Take 2 hours before eating.

   b. Sit or lie down for 30 minutes after taking a dose.

   c. Take with a full glass of water.

   d. Take the vitamin after getting out of bed every morning.

3. A thiamine deficiency is most likely to develop in which of the following groups?

   a. alcoholics

   b. preschoolers

   c. senior citizens

   d. teenagers

4. You work in an emergency room in a large hospital in a major city. A client presents with erythematous skin sores, gastrointestinal (GI) complaints, headaches, and dizziness. The physician suspects pellagra. You will administer which of the following?

   a. pyridoxine (B_6)

   b. pantothenic (B_5)

   c. thiamine (B_1)

   d. niacin (B_3)

5. Your client, a 53-year-old male, has been diagnosed with pernicious anemia. You have just given him his first injection of vitamin B12. He asks you why he can't take pills instead. Your response should be:

   a. "The oral form of vitamin B_{12} is more costly than the injectable form."

   b. "You would have to sit upright for 30 minutes after an oral dose of B_{12} to decrease esophageal irritation."

   c. "The oral form of B_{12} is too irritating to the lining of the stomach."

   d. "Oral forms of vitamin B_{12} are not absorbed from the GI tract."

6. Your client is complaining of signs and symptoms of peripheral neuritis. Which of the following vitamin preparations should she be taking?

   a. B_1

   b. B_3

   c. B_6

   d. B_{12}

7. A client is taking cyanocobalamin (Nascobal) for a nutritional deficiency. A nurse would caution use of the drug if which of the following were present:

   a. rhinitis

   b. high blood pressure

   c. fever

   d. headache

8. You are discussing healthy lifestyles with a group of residents at a retirement complex. One resident asks you which vitamin can help prevent cancer. Your response would be:

   a. "Vitamin B_{12} helps prevent all types of cancer."

   b. "Vitamins A and C help prevent certain types of cancer."

   c. "Folic acid is helpful in the prevention of cancer."

   d. "Vitamins don't help prevent cancer."

9. You have a client who takes several vitamins, herbs, and dietary supplements. She tells you she takes a double dose of vitamin C every day. You are aware that she could be at risk for:

   a. kidney stones

   b. dry, itchy skin

   c. increased blood pressure

   d. severe headaches

10. When teaching a client about dietary folic acid deficiency anemia, you will advise him to:

    a. increase the amount of cooked fruit and vegetables to his diet

    b. add an extra serving of meat each day to his diet

    c. add one glass of fruit juice to his diet daily

    d. decrease the amount of dairy products he consumes each day

CHAPTER 32

Minerals and Electrolytes

■ Exercises

Fill in the blank.

1. _____ occur in the body in ionic form.

2. Electrically charged particles in the body are called _____.

3. Electrolytes maintain _____ balance of body fluids.

4. Minerals that are required in large amounts in the body are called _____.

5. Minerals that are required in small amounts in body are _____ or _____ _____.

Match the following.

1. ____ deferoxamine (Desferal)

2. ____ succimer (Chemet)

3. ____ magnesium sulfate

4. ____ sodium bicarbonate

5. ____ Pedialyte

6. ____ ferrous sulfate (Feosol)

7. ____ penicillamine (Cuprimine)

8. ____ potassium chloride (KCL)

9. ____ selenium

10. ____ sodium polystyrene sulfonate (Kayexalate)

a. Cation exchange resin used in treatment of hyperkalemia

b. Removes excess copper in clients with Wilson's disease

c. Prototype for iron preparations

d. Used in treating hypokalemia

e. Used to treat metabolic acidosis

f. Depresses central nervous system and smooth, skeletal, and cardiac muscles

g. Chelating agent for iron

h. Oral electrolyte solution used to treat diarrhea in children

i. Used to treat lead poisoning in children

j. Dietary supplement used as an antioxidant

Fill in the chart.

Imbalance	Cause	Signs and symptoms
Hyperkalemia		
Hypochloremia metabolic alkalosis		
Hypernatremia		
Hyponatremia		
Hypokalemia		
Hyperchloremia metabolic acidosis		
Hypomagnesemia		
Hypermagnesemia		

■ Clinical Challenge

A client is admitted to the emergency room with the following signs and symptoms: weakness, lethargy, drowsiness, muscle weakness, abdominal distention, and decreased blood pressure. Lab work including an electrocardiogram (ECG) is ordered. Your assessment reveals that the client is 69 years old and has had vomiting and diarrhea for a week. He takes Digoxin, Lasix, "a blood pressure pill," and a multivitamin. Lab reports reveal: serum potassium level 2.9 mEq/L; serum creatinine 2.1 mg/dL; serum blood urea nitrogen 25 mg/dL; and serum glucose level 186. ECG changes indicate depressed ST segment, inverted T wave, and prolonged P-R interval. From the assessment data, what medical diagnosis do you suspect? Describe the nursing care for this client.

■ Review Questions

1. Your client has hemochromatosis. The physician prescribes deferoxamine (Desferal). It is important for the client to understand that:

   a. he must increase fluids while taking the medication

   b. he should take the medication on an empty stomach

   c. his urine will be reddish brown

   d. his blood pressure may increase slightly

2. A client's father has Wilson's disease. Which of the following drugs can he take prophylactically for this condition?

   a. deferoxamine (Desferal)

   b. succimer (Chemet)

   c. penicillamine (Cuprimine)

   d. sodium polystyrene sulfonate (Kayexalate)

3. A 5-year-old is admitted to the hospital with a serum iron level of 55 µg/100mL. Succimer (Chemet) therapy is started. The nurse will expect which of the following adverse effects?

   a. anorexia

   b. headache

   c. joint pain

   d. sore throat

4. Magnesium sulfate is indicated for a 35-year-old pregnant woman with eclampsia. Before administration, consideration will given to which of the following?

   a. hepatic disease

   b. chronic obstructive pulmonary disease

   c. renal disease

   d. cardiotoxicity

5. Your client is admitted to the hospital with dehydration. According to the following lab values, which electrolyte imbalance is she experiencing? (serum sodium 115 mEq/L; serum chloride 100 mEq/L; serum potassium 3.5 mEq/L.)

   a. hyperchloremia

   b. hyperkalemia

   c. hyponatremia

   d. hypokalemia

6. Your client is receiving magnesium sulfate for eclampsia. Which of the following IV preparations would you have on hand if she began to experience lethargy, skeletal muscle weakness, decreased blood pressure, and respiratory distress?

   a. Narcan

   b. calcium gluconate

   c. KCL

   d. magnesium oxide

7. Your client, a 42-year-old female, has been started on ferrous sulfate (Feosol) for iron deficiency anemia. Which of the following instructions should be given to her?

   a. "Ferrous sulfate should be taken at night."

   b. "You will need to take the iron preparation for about 2 months."

   c. "You may take a drug holiday once a week."

   d. "Take the medication on an empty stomach if you can tolerate the gastric irritation."

8. Which of the following lab values indicate metabolic acidosis?

   a. pH 7.20 and bicarbonate 78 mEq/L

   b. pH 7.57 and bicarbonate 30 mEq/L

   c. pH 7.4 and bicarbonate 24 mEq/L

   d. pH 7.6 and bicarbonate 28 mEq/L

9. Your client has been diagnosed with hypokalemia. She insists on getting out of bed and walking to the bathroom by herself. An appropriate nursing diagnosis for her would be:

   a. risk for injury

   b. activity intolerance

   c. impaired bed mobility

   d. noncompliance

10. You are teaching a group of third graders about the use of fluoride supplements. Which of the following would you include in your presentation?

    a. "Swish the solution around in your mouth once and swallow."

    b. "Swish the solution several times in your mouth and spit out."

    c. "Mix the solution with a full glass of water and swallow."

    d. "Rinse with fluoride preparation after each meal."

CHAPTER 33

General Characteristics of Antimicrobial Drugs

■ Exercises

Match the following.

1. ____ anaerobic bacteria
2. ____ viruses
3. ____ *Escherichia coli*
4. ____ nosocomial infection
5. ____ streptococci
6. ____ aerobic bacteria
7. ____ pathogenic
8. ____ "opportunistic" microorganism
9. ____ bactericidal
10. ____ fungi

a. Intracellular parasites that survive only in living tissue
b. Bacteria that require oxygen
c. Normal endogenous or environmental flora
d. An infection acquired in a hospital
e. Plant-like organisms that live as parasites on living tissue
f. A drug that kills a microorganism
g. Normal microbial skin flora
h. Disease-producing
i. An organism that most often causes urinary tract infections
j. Bacteria that cannot live in the presence of oxygen

Complete the chart by placing a check mark in the appropriate column.

Bacteria pathogen	Gram-positive; gram-negative	Normal body flora	Medical conditions
E. coli			
Enterococci			
Staphylococcus spp.			
Bacteroides spp.			
Klebsiella spp.			
Streptococcus spp.			
Proteus spp.			

Answer the following.

1. List the major defense mechanisms of the body.

2. List contributing factors for the increasing prevalence of antibiotic-resistant microorganisms.

3. List the mechanisms of action for antimicrobial drugs.

■Review Questions

1. It is important to administer antimicrobial drugs at scheduled, evenly spaced intervals to ensure:
   a. use of all packaged medication
   b. therapeutic blood levels
   c. minimal adverse effects
   d. client compliance

2. Which of the following outcomes would be appropriate for a client receiving antimicrobial therapy who has a wound infection?
   a. decrease in white blood cell count
   b. increase in malaise and lethargy
   c. increase in drainage
   d. decrease in appetite

3. Most intravenous administration of antimicrobial drugs should infuse over:
   a. 5 to 10 minutes
   b. 15 to 30 minutes
   c. 30 to 60 minutes
   d. 60 to 90 minutes

4. Which of the following adverse effects will occur with most antimicrobial agents?
   a. diarrhea
   b. nausea
   c. headache
   d. hypersensitivity

5. You have an order to mix an antibiotic with multivitamins in 50 cc of solution and administer intravenously over 1 hour. Which of the following nursing measures is most appropriate?
   a. Prepare and administer the order as written.
   b. Check with the head nurse before administration of the IV medications.

c. Call the physician to clarify the order.
   d. Decrease the amount of solution used to mix the antibiotic powder because the multivitamins will be added to the antibiotics.

6. A client has been receiving antimicrobial therapy for 2 weeks. He has lost 7 pounds during that time. When the nurse questions him concerning the weight loss, he tells her he doesn't feel like eating. The most appropriate nursing diagnosis for this client would be:
   a. fatigue related to infection
   b. deficient knowledge: use of antimicrobial drugs
   c. imbalanced nutrition: less than body requirements related to adverse effects of drug therapy
   d. risk for injury: related to adverse drug effects

7. The most effective method of preventing infection is:
   a. accurate administration of antibiotics
   b. the use of isolation procedures
   c. keeping skin clean and dry
   d. handwashing

8. If severe adverse effects of antimicrobial therapy occur, clients should:
   a. stop the drug immediately
   b. continue taking the medication until it is all gone
   c. report adverse effects to health care provider
   d. decrease the dosage and continue therapy

9. Which of the following laboratory tests identifies infectious agents by measuring the titer in the serum of a diseased host?
   a. Gram's stain
   b. culture
   c. serology
   d. detection of antigens

10. The duration for antimicrobial therapy is usually:
    a. 3 to 5 days
    b. 7 to 10 days
    c. 12 to 15 days
    d. 14 to 21 days

CHAPTER 34

Beta-Lactam Antibacterials: Penicillins, Cephalosporins, and Others

■ Exercises

Answer the following.

1. List four groups of beta-lactam antibiotics.

2. Describe the mechanism of action for beta-lactam antibacterial drugs.

3. Explain how a beta-lactamase inhibitor, when combined with a penicillin, produces a therapeutic effect.

4. Why might some clients be allergic to both penicillins and cephalosporins?

5. List adverse effects of penicillins.

Match the following.

1. ____ amoxicillin (Amoxil)

2. ____ nafcillin (Unipen)

3. ____ cephalosporins

4. ____ cefoxitin (Mefoxin)

5. ____ penicillin G

6. ____ aztreonam (Azactam)

7. ____ ampicillin

8. ____ imipenem/cilastatin (Primaxin)

9. ____ penicillin V

10. ____ carbenicillin

a. An extended-spectrum/antipseudomonal penicillin used to treat urinary tract infections and prostatitis

b. Active against *Bacteroides fragilis*, an anaerobic organism resistant to most drugs

c. Administered only by the oral route

d. A monobactam active against gram-negative bacteria

e. A broad-spectrum, semisynthetic penicillin used for gram-negative and gram-positive bacterial infections

f. A carbapenem that requires lidocaine to be added for an IM injection to decrease pain

g. Penicillinase-resistant penicillin

h. Broad-spectrum antibacterial agents that come from fungus

i. Prototype for penicillins

j. An aminopenicillin that is converted to ampicillin in the body

Place T (true) or F(false) in each blank.

1. ____ Beta-lactam antibiotics are most effective when bacterial cells are dividing.

2. ____ The most serious adverse effect of the penicillins is nephropathy.

3. ____ Penicillins are more effective in infections caused by gram-negative bacteria.

4. ____ An allergic reaction to one penicillin usually means a client will be allergic to all penicillins.

5. ____ In general, cephalosporins are more active against gram-positive organisms.

6. ____ Third-generation cephalosporins are used to treat meningeal infections.

7. ____ Penicillins are more effective in most streptococcal and staphylococcal infections.

8. ____ Penicillin is the most common cause of drug-induced anaphylaxis.

9. ____ Second-generation cephalosporins are often used for surgical prophylaxis with prosthetic implants.

10. ____ In the hospital setting, the intramuscular route is always used for the administration of penicillin.

■ Clinical Challenge

Your client is an 11-year-old male who has a positive throat culture for streptococci. He is given a prescription for amoxicillin capsules 250 mg every 8 hours PO for 10 days. What should your teaching plan include? What should you tell the client and his mother about taking the medication at school?

■ Review Questions

1. A 28-year-old female has been given a prescription for cefdinir (Omnicef) 300 mg every 12 hours for bronchitis. Which of the following statements by her indicates that she has an understanding of cefdinir therapy?

   a. "I take my medication on an empty stomach."

   b. "I take my medication every 4 hours."

   c. "I take my antibiotic right before breakfast and before my evening meal."

   d. "I will take this medication as long as my throat hurts."

2. A client is 73 years old and is taking a cephalosporin. There is a possibility that this client may develop:

   a. nephrotoxicity

   b. pernicious anemia

   c. fibromyalgia

   d. endocarditis

3. When explaining to your client that he should not drink cranberry or orange juice while taking Nafcillin, you will advise him that:

   a. if acidic juices are ingested, solid foods should be taken with penicillin

   b. oral penicillins are destroyed by acids

   c. acids increase the absorption rate of penicillins

   d. acids increase the blood level of penicillins

4. Imipenem (Primaxin) is contraindicated in clients with:

   a. anemia

   b. hypertension

   c. diabetes mellitus

   d. seizure disorders

5. While instructing new RN graduates about the use of penicillin and an aminoglycoside, the following should be included:

   a. When giving an IM injection, draw up the penicillin first, then the aminoglycoside.

   b. Give each drug in separate syringes if administering IM.

   c. Never mix the two in a syringe or IV solution.

   d. The two are not prescribed to be given at the same time.

6. Which of the following electrolyte imbalances may occur with the use of large doses of IV penicillin G potassium?

    a. hypokalemia

    b. hyperkalemia

    c. hyponatremia

    d. hypernatremia

7. Your client has cancer of both kidneys. Which of the following will be important in determining the correct dosage of a cephalosporin?

    a. urinary output

    b. creatinine clearance level

    c. 24-hour urine

    d. urine pH

8. When teaching a young mother about administration of a penicillin, the home care nurse will advise:

    a. shaking the liquid suspension to resuspend the medication before giving it

    b. warming the medication prior to administration

    c. administering with a fruit juice

    d. giving only when the child is awake

9. You are the medication nurse for an 8-hour shift. You must give ampicillin IM. In planning for preparation of all the medications on the floor that you will be giving, you are aware that reconstituted ampicillin must be given:

    a. with breakfast

    b. within 15 minutes of preparation

    c. in the deltoid muscle

    d. within 1 hour of preparation

10. Your client is taking a cephalosporin for a urinary tract infection. Which of the following drugs would you inform your client that he should not take with the cephalosporin therapy?

    a. Lanoxin

    b. Mylanta

    c. erythromycin

    d. Valium

CHAPTER 35

Aminoglycosides and Fluoroquinolones

■ Exercises

Fill in the blank.

1. Aminoglycosides are bactericidal agents used to treat infections caused by gram- _____ microorganisms.

2. Aminoglycosides accumulate in high concentrations in the _____ and _____ _____.

3. In pseudomonal infections, aminoglycosides can be given with _____.

4. _____ and _____ may be used in the treatment of hepatic coma.

5. _____ is used in the treatment of intestinal amebiasis.

6. _____ is not recommended for use in infants and children.

7. Dosages of animoglycosides are adjusted according to serum drug levels and _____ _____.

8. Fluoroquinolones are used for infections caused by aerobic gram-_____ microorganisms.

9. _____ decrease the effects of fluoroquinolones.

10. Do not take _____ with food.

Place T (true) or F (false) in each blank.

1. ____ Nephrotoxicity occurs more often with fluoroquinolones than with aminoglycosides.

2. ____ Many nosocomial infections are caused by gram-negative organisms.

3. ____ Fluoroquinolones are contraindicated in children younger than 18 years of age.

4. ____ Smaller doses of aminoglycosides are indicated for urinary tract infections.

5. ____ Aminoglycosides should be given no longer than 14 days.

6. ____ If nephrotoxicity occurs with aminoglycoside therapy, it is reversible when the drug is discontinued.

7. ____ Hepatic impairment is not a factor in aminoglycoside therapy.

8. ____ Trough blood levels should be drawn 30 to 60 minutes after administering a drug.

9. ____ Ciprofloxacin (Cipro) must be taken 1 hour before or 2 hours after a meal.

10. ____ Oral fluoroquinolones can cause dizziness or light headedness.

■ Clinical Challenge

Your client is being treated with ciprofloxacin (Cipro) for gonorrhea. What assessment data are needed before therapy is started? What instructions will you give to the client?

■ Review Questions

1. Your client is to start on tobramycin (Nebcin) for a nosocomial infection. Which of the following would be the most helpful in determining the correct dosage of Nebcin?

   a. the client's blood pressure

   b. the client's weight

   c. what time the client eats breakfast

   d. other client medication

2. Clients who are on aminoglycoside therapy would be assessed for factors that could predispose to:

   a. cardiotoxicity and hepatotoxicity

   b. diabetes mellitus and nephrotoxicity

   c. ototoxicity and hypertension

   d. nephrotoxicity and ototoxicity

3. Your client has been on ciprofloxacin (Cipro) for acute sinusitis for 10 days. Which of the following laboratory tests should be initiated?

   a. complete blood count

   b. blood glucose level

   c. prothrombin time

   d. electrocardiogram (ECG)

4. A client is taking norfloxacin (Noroxin) for a urinary tract infection. The nurse will be sure to include the following when discussing norfloxacin therapy:

   a. Take with meals.

   b. Sunscreen lotions do not prevent photosensitivity reactions.

   c. Limit fluid intake to 1 quart per day.

   d. PO medication is taken once a day.

5. Gentamicin (Garamycin) is begun for your client. Which laboratory value should be monitored?

   a. potassium level

   b. serum creatinine level

   c. serum albumin level

   d. prothrombin time

6. Neomycin has been ordered for your client. You will administer this drug by which of the following routes?

   a. oral

   b. subcutaneous

   c. intramuscular

   d. intravenous

7. Your client is taking gentamicin. A trough level should be obtained:

   a. 15 to 30 minutes before the next dose

   b. 1 hour before the next dose

   c. 2 hours before the next dose

   d. 30 minutes after the next dose

8. Your client, age 50, has been receiving gentamicin therapy for 3 days. Which of the following would be the most appropriate nursing action?

   a. monitoring blood pressure

   b. assessing for tinnitus

   c. monitoring weight

   d. assessing for gout

9. Your client has completed a 7-day course of ciprofloxacin (Cipro). She tells you that she thinks she has a vaginal yeast infection. You suspect that she has:

   a. a suprainfection

   b. an allergic reaction

   c. a sexually transmitted disease

   d. a skin disease

10. Your client has been taking ciprofloxacin (Cipro) for 3 days for pneumonia. She calls the clinic and reports that she has an itchy rash all over her body. You advise her to:

    a. stop taking the drug immediately

    b. request a topical cream for the rash

    c. decrease the dosage of Cipro

    d. continue the drug as ordered

CHAPTER 36

Tetracyclines, Sulfonamides, and Urinary Agents

■Exercises

Answer the following.

1. List four clinical indications for tetracyclines.

2. Describe the mechanism of action for tetracyclines.

3. Describe the mechanism of action for sulfonamides.

4. Why are tetracyclines contraindicated in pregnant women and children up to 8 years of age?

5. Outline a teaching plan for a client who has a urinary tract infection.

Place T (true) or F (false) in each blank.

1. ____ Tetracyclines may be substituted for penicillin in treating streptococcal pharyngitis.

2. ____ Tetracyclines should not be substituted for penicillin in serious staphylococcal infections.

3. ____ Once resistance to one sulfonamide develops, cross-resistance to others is common.

4. ____ Urinary antiseptics can be used to treat urinary tract infections and ulcerative colitis.

5. ____ Doxycycline can be used in clients with renal failure.

6. ____ The intramuscular route is preferred for tetracycline therapy.

7. ____ With sulfonamide therapy, alkaline urine decreases drug solubility.

8. ____ Urine pH must be acidic for Mandelamine therapy to be therapeutic.

9. ____ Sulfonamides may be used to treat urinary tract infections in children older than 2 months.

10. ____ Nausea is an allergic response to Bactrim.

■ Clinical Challenge

A client comes to the clinic complaining of signs and symptoms of a urinary tract infection. After a thorough assessment, you determine that the client is allergic to penicillin and "sulfur" drugs. The nurse indicates the allergies on the client's chart. A urinalysis does indicate that the client has a urinary tract infection. The physician orders sulfamethoxazole, trimethoprim, sulfamethoxazole (Bactrim). What should the nurse do?

■ Review Questions

1. Your client, age 19, has been on tetracycline therapy for 3 years. Which of the following should be monitored?

   a. blood pressure

   b. liver function

   c. blood glucose level

   d. renal function

2. A 58-year-old female is being started on sulfonamide therapy for ulcerative colitis. Which of the following would be an appropriate outcome for this client?

   a. urinary output of 100 to 250 mL daily

   b. urinary output of 250 to 500 mL daily

   c. urinary output of 600 1000 mL daily

   d. urinary output of 1200 to 1500 mL daily

3. Which of the following statements by your client indicates that she does not have an understanding of doxycycline (Vibramycin) therapy?

   a. "I will be spending my summer at the beach."

   b. "I will take my medication by mouth."

   c. "If I experience perineal itching, I will let my doctor know."

   d. "I take my medication with saltine crackers."

4. When instructing a client concerning tetracycline therapy, which of the following should be included in your teaching plan?

   a. The intramuscular route is preferred.

   b. Avoid dairy product ingestion with tetracycline.

   c. Outdated tetracycline may be used up to 1 year.

   d. Always take all tetracycline on an empty stomach.

5. Which of the following drugs is used as prophylaxis for recurrent urinary tract infections?

   a. nitrofurantoin (Macrodantin)

   b. trimethoprim (Trimpex)

   c. fosfomycin (Monurol)

   d. mafenide (Sulfamylon)

6. A 30-year-old female comes to the clinic complaining of dysuria, burning, and frequency and urgency of urination. A urinalysis indicates she has a urinary tract infection. The physician prescribes sulfamethoxazole (Gantanol). Which of the following drugs may also be prescribed to relieve her discomfort?

   a. methenamine mandelate (Mandelamine)

   b. phenazopyridine (Pyridium)

   c. fosfomycin (Monurol)

   d. sulfamethizole (Thiosulfil)

7. Your client is being treated for Rocky Mountain Spotted fever. He is taking tetracycline (Achromycin) 2 gm/day in 4 equal doses. He complains of soreness and white patches in his mouth, and states that his tongue has turned black. You suspect that:

   a. his condition has worsened

   b. he has a monilial superinfection

   c. he is having adverse effects from the Achromycin

   d. he is having an allergic reaction to a food substance

8. Your client will be taking sulfamethoxazole, trimethoprim (Bactrim) for an extended period of time. Which of the following laboratory tests would *not* be included in periodic clinic visits?

   a. aspartate aminotransferase levels

   b. blood urea nitrogen

   c. pulmonary function

   d. hematuria

9. A client is to be placed on sulfonamide therapy for a urinary tract infection. Which of the following drugs being taken by the client should be reported to the client's physician?

    a. Fosamax

    b. aspirin

    c. Synthroid

    d. Inderal

10. The client is taking fosfomycin (Monurol) for a urinary tract infection. The nurse is aware that administration of this drug is:

    a. without food

    b. with a full glass of water

    c. immediately after the powder is mixed with water

    d. three times a day

CHAPTER 37

Macrolides and Miscellaneous Antibacterials

■ Exercises

Match the following.

1. ____ telithromycin (Ketek)

2. ____ chloramphenicol (Chloromycetin)

3. ____ azithromycin (Zithromax)

4. ____ clindamycin hydrochloride (Cleocin)

5. ____ metronidazole (Flagyl)

6. ____ quinupristin/dalfopristin (Synercid)

7. ____ spectinomycin (Trobicin)

8. ____ linezolid (Zyrox)

9. ____ erythromycin

10. ____ vancomycin

a. Used to treat urethritis and cervicitis

b. Myelosuppression may result from use

c. Macrolide prototype

d. Effective against trichomoniasis

e. Used to treat infections caused by *Bacteriodes fragilis*

f. A streptogramin antimicrobial

g. Used to treat severe infections

h. Used to treat gonococcal exposure

i. New drug that will treat *Streptococcus pneumoniae* infections

j. Used to treat serious infections for which no adequate substitute drug is available

Place T (true) or F (false) in each blank.

1. ____ The rapid infusion of vancomycin, which causes flushing, is referred to as the "red man effect."

2. ____ Azithromycin (Zithromax) should be taken with food.

3. ____ Clarithromycin (Biaxin) may be taken without regard to meals.

4. ____ Macrolides should be taken with 6 to 8 oz of water.

5. ____ Vancomycin should not be given to children under 18 years of age.

6. ____ Vancomycin is given orally to treat pseudomembranous colitis.

7. ____ Clarithromycin (Biaxin) decreases carbamazepine levels.

8. ____ Therapeutic levels of chloramphenicol (Chloromycetin) are 10 to 20 mcg/mL.

9. ____ Trobicin is given to prevent gram-positive infections in clients who are at risk for methicillin-resistant *Staphylococcus aureus* infections.

10. ____ Flagyl is effective against *Clostridium* spp.

■ Clinical Challenge

Your client is a 52-year-old female who has peritonitis. She has been taking clindamycin hydrochloride (Cleocin) 300 mg PO every 6 hours for 5 days. She reports fever and severe diarrhea with pus and blood. What do you suspect? What do you tell her?

She asks you how she got this infection when she was already taking an antibiotic. How do you respond? What will be her treatment plan?

■ Review Questions

1. Your client is to receive clindamycin (Cleocin). In order to promote therapeutic effects, you will administer the drug:
   a. with a fruit juice
   b. with a light snack
   c. when client has an empty stomach
   d. with meals

2. Linezolid (Zyvox) is being given to your client for pneumonia. He has been told that he should decrease his salt intake. You will monitor his:
   a. blood glucose level
   b. weight
   c. blood urea nitrogen level
   d. blood pressure

3. Your client has *Haemophilus* meningitis. He is allergic to penicillin and has been placed on chloramphenicol. He should be closely monitored for:
   a. diabetes mellitus
   b. blood dyscrasia
   c. hepatic toxicity
   d. ototoxicity

4. Erythromycin has been prescribed for a client. Which of the following may have been considered when selecting this drug?
   a. age
   b. diet
   c. activity level
   d. family history

5. Erythromycin can interfere with the elimination of other drugs. Which of the following explains why toxicity of the other drugs may occur?
   a. The affected drugs are eliminated more slowly, increasing their serum levels.
   b. The affected drugs are eliminated very quickly, decreasing their serum levels.
   c. Erythromycin causes an increase in metabolism of the other drugs.
   d. Erythromycin can cause an antagonistic effect when given with other drugs.

6. Your client is receiving IV erythromycin lactobionate for bacterial endocarditis. After 6 hours of therapy, he complains of burning pain and is warm at the IV infusion site. Which of the following would be your *initial* action?
   a. Change infusion site every 48 to 72 hours.
   b. Slow the rate of infusion.
   c. Apply an ice compress.
   d. Discontinue the IV.

7. Your client is receiving linezolid (Zyvox). Which of the following foods should he avoid?
   a. green beans
   b. blue cheese
   c. beets
   d. red meat

8. Your client is having colorectal surgery and is receiving metronidazole (Flagyl) for prevention of anaerobic bacterial infections. You should monitor him for which of the following serious adverse effects?
   a. migraine headache
   b. seizures
   c. increased blood pressure
   d. confusion

9. In a client receiving clarithromycin (Biaxin), which of the following lab values should be monitored in relation to dosage?
   a. creatinine clearance
   b. prothrombin time
   c. liver enzymes
   d. urine specific gravity

10. Your client has a severe systemic infection and is being treated with vancomycin IV. You will monitor the client for:
    a. decrease in blood pressure and flushing
    b. increase in fever and heart rate
    c. shortness of breath and dizziness
    d. increase in blood pressure and itching

CHAPTER 38

Drugs for Tuberculosis and *Mycobacterium Avium* Complex (MAC) Disease

■ Exercises

Answer the following.

1. Describe the physiological action of isoniazid (INH).

2. Differentiate latent tuberculosis infection (LTBI) from active tuberculosis (TB).

3. What is a major concern among public health care providers concerning tuberculosis?

4. How can nurses help control the spread of TB?

5. Name five primary drugs used to treat TB.

Match the following.

1. ____ rifampin (Rifadin)

2. ____ pyrazinamide

3. ____ capreomycin (Capastat)

4. ____ isoniazid (INH)

5. ____ ofloxacin

6. ____ streptomycin

7. ____ rifabutin (Mycobutin)

8. ____ ethambutol (Myambutol)

9. ____ rifapentine (Priftin)

10. ____ Rifater

a. Used to treat pulmonary tuberculosis; less frequent administration than rifampin

b. An antitubercular drug that inhibits synthesis of ribonucleic acid and interferes with mycobacterial protein metabolism

c. Synergistic in combination with isoniazid (INH) to kill tuberculosis bacilli

d. Used with INH and rifampin for the first 2 months of active tuberculosis treatment

e. Used in a combination of INH, rifampin, and pyrazinamide to promote compliance of drug therapy for tuberculosis

f. A fluoroquinolone that can be used to treat multidrug-resistant tuberculosis in adults

g. Most commonly used antitubercular drug

h. A drug that has tuberculostatic properties and may be used in combination with other drugs for treatment

i. An aminoglycoside antibiotic used in a medication regimen for tuberculosis

j. Used in clients with HIV who have *Mycobacterium avium* complex and as a substitute for rifampin.

Place T (true) or F (false) in each blank.

1. ____ Older adults are more likely to have prominent signs and symptoms of tuberculosis than younger adults.

2. ____ Initial signs and symptoms of tuberculosis in children may occur within a few weeks of exposure.

3. ____ Pyrazinamide is contraindicated during pregnancy.

4. ____ INH therapy should be once a week.

5. ____ Screening for tuberculosis is done only at public health departments.

6. ____ People with silicosis are more likely to have TB.

7. ____ Hepatitis is more likely to occur during the first 8 weeks of INH therapy.

8. ____ INH therapy is questioned in older adults, due to the increased risk of drug-induced hepatotoxicity.

9. ____ Rifampin increases blood levels and therapeutic effects of anti-HIV drugs.

10. ____ INH increases blood levels of phenytoin (Dilantin).

■ Clinical Challenge

You are a home health nurse, and you are planning a visit to a 78-year-old Hispanic female who lives with her daughter and son-in-law, and their four children. Your client has active TB and has just returned home after 2 weeks in the hospital. What do you plan for your first home visit?

■ Review Questions

1. Your client, age 43, has been diagnosed with active tuberculosis. He is taking multiple drug therapy, including INH and rifampin (Rifadin). Which of the following laboratory tests should be done at least once a month?

   a. serum alanine, aspartate aminotransferases (ALT and AST), and bilirubin

   b. red blood count, white blood count, and differential

   c. thyroid-stimulating hormone, thyroxine, and triiodothyronine levels

   d. fasting blood sugar and 2-hour postprandial blood sugar

2. INH therapy has been started on your client. You have completed a thorough assessment. Of the following prescribed drugs for the client, which one should be reported to the client's physician?

   a. acetaminophen (Tylenol)

   b. vitamin B_6

   c. diltiazem hydrochloride (Cardizem)

   d. folic acid

3. When teaching clients concerning the use of antituberculosis drugs, a nurse would advise which of the following?

   a. There is no need for concern of liver damage.

   b. Drug therapy for tuberculosis is a lifetime commitment.

   c. Drug therapy lasts only a couple of months.

   d. Hypersensitivity reactions are more likely to occur between the third and eighth week of drug therapy.

4. A 28-year-old female is being treated for active TB with INH and rifampin (Rifadin). She should be informed that:

   a. she should have her blood glucose levels checked at least every month while on drug therapy

   b. she should use additional birth control if she is taking an oral contraceptive

   c. she will probably gain weight while on TB drug therapy

   d. she will most likely have to take the medication for 2 to 3 years

5. Your client who has active TB asks you how long it will take the medication to make him feel better. An appropriate response would be:

   a. "Don't worry about that. You are going to feel better soon."

   b. "You will probably be on the medication for about a year."

   c. "You should begin to feel better within 2 to 3 weeks of starting the medications."

   d. "That's really hard to predict."

6. Which of the following groups of people who may be on INH therapy are more likely to have serious liver impairment?

   a. Asians

   b. alcoholics

   c. diabetics

   d. homeless

7. Why should rifampin therapy not be used in people with HIV?

   a. Rifampin increases the severity of the anti-HIV drugs' adverse effects.

   b. Rifampin increases blood levels and therapeutic effects of anti-HIV drugs.

   c. Rifampin's therapeutic effects are decreased by the anti-HIV drugs.

   d. Rifampin decreases blood levels and therapeutic effects of anti-HIV drugs.

8. Your client has recently been diagnosed with active TB and is taking INH and rifampin. Pyrazinamide is also added for the first 2 months of therapy. Which of the following laboratory tests should be done during the first 2 months of therapy in relation to pyrazinamide?

   a. blood urea nitrogen levels

   b. uric acid levels

   c. creatinine levels

   d. urine osmolality

9. A client is receiving ethambutol as part of a four-drug regimen for TB. Which of the following may be of concern for this client?

   a. driving his car in town

   b. eating a high protein, low-fat diet

   c. playing tennis every weekend

   d. smoking a pack of cigarettes per day

10. Your client is taking rifampin (Rifadin) for active TB. When discussing this drug with the client, you should stress that:

    a. the drug does not cause gastrointestinal upset

    b. the drug can cause seizures

    c. a "butterfly rash" may appear across the face but will go away once therapy is concluded

    d. the red/orange discoloration of urine is a side effect but is harmless

CHAPTER 39

Antiviral Drugs

■ Exercises

Fill in the blanks using the following words. Some words may be used more than once.

granulocytopenia   acyclovir
ribavirin   valganciclovir
Kaletra   viruses
zidovudine   ganciclovir
vidarabine   trifluridine
tenofovir   ritonavir
parasites   amantadine
valacyclovir   amprenavir
thrombocytopenia   rimantadine
famciclovir   antibodies

1. Viruses are intracellular _____ that live and replicate inside body cells.

2. _____ cause _____ to be produced in the body.

3. _____, _____, and _____ are used to treat herpes simplex and herpes zoster infections.

4. _____ is used to treat immunocompromised clients who have herpes simplex infections.

5. _____ and _____ treat recurrent genital herpes.

6. _____ and _____ are used to prevent cytomegalovirus infections in clients with organ transplants or HIV infections.

7. Ganciclovir causes _____ and _____.

8. _____ and _____ are used topically to treat keratoconjunctivitis and corneal ulcers caused by herpes simplex.

9. _____ is the prototype of nucleoside reverse transcriptase inhibitors (NRTIs).

10. _____ has been used to treat hepatitis B.

11. _____ can increase sedation and respiratory depression when used with benzodiazepines.

12. _____ is a sulfonamide and contains high concentrations of vitamin E.

13. _____ is a combination of ritonavir and lopinavir.

14. _____ and _____ are used to prevent and treat influenza A.

15. _____ is used to treat bronchiolitis.

Answer the following.

1. List "constitutional symptoms" of acute viral infections.

2. List the four classes of drugs used for HIV infection and AIDS.

3. List common side effects of drugs used to treat influenza A.

4. Why are herbal products not recommended during use of antiretroviral medications?

5. How do antiviral drugs produce a therapeutic action?

■ Clinical Challenge

Your client is a 23-year-old female who has just been diagnosed with HIV. She is to start on zidovudine and ritonavir. She is extremely upset and keeps saying she cannot believe this is happening to her. How do you approach her concerning drug therapy? What specific instructions do you give her concerning these drugs?

■ Review Questions

1. Your client is a 42-year-old male who was recently diagnosed with AIDS. He is to begin drug therapy with zidovudine (AZT) 300 mg PO. You will anticipate which of the following dosage schedules?

   a. every 4 hours

   b. twice a day

   c. three times a day

   d. four times a day

2. A client who takes abacavir (Ziagen) should avoid taking the drug with:

   a. high-protein meals

   b. fatty foods

   c. acidic fruit juices

   d. high-carbohydrate foods

3. Your client who has been taking zidovudine (AZT) for 3 weeks is complaining of numbness, burning, and pain in his hands and feet. You suspect that his physician will:

   a. continue therapy as prescribed

   b. decrease the dosage of AZT

   c. add a therapeutic dose of acetaminophen daily

   d. discontinue AZT and prescribe another antiretroviral drug

4. A client is diagnosed with AIDS and has developed cytomegalovirus infections. He is placed on ganciclovir therapy. When discussing the drug therapy with the client, you stress that thrombocytopenia may occur:

   a. during the first 2 weeks of therapy

   b. during the first month of therapy

   c. at the end of therapy

   d. years after the therapy has been stopped

5. A 70-year-old male has developed keratoconjunctivitis caused by herpes simplex virus. Trifluridine has been prescribed. The health care provider is aware that the drug:

   a. regimen will last at least 6 weeks

   b. is given orally

   c. should not be used longer than 21 days

   d. does not have adverse effects

6. Before clients are placed on amprenavir (Agenerase), they should be assessed for an allergic reaction to which of the following drugs?

   a. penicillins

   b. sulfonamides

   c. benzodiazepines

   d. acetaminophens

7. Your client has been diagnosed with influenza A, and amantadine (Symmetrel) has been prescribed for her. You will inform her of which of the following side effects?

   a. nausea

   b. headache

   c. palpitations

   d. burning sensation in hands and feet

8. Which of the following drugs is given for prevention of influenza in children?

    a. amantadine (Symmetrel)

    b. zanamivir (Relenza)

    c. oseltamivir (Tamiflu)

    d. rimantadine (Flumadine)

9. A client who has AIDS is taking cidofovir (Vistide) for treatment of cytomegalovirus retinitis. Which of the following should be monitored?

    a. serum creatinine

    b. hematocrit

    c. uric acid

    d. blood glucose

10. Your client is taking an antiretroviral drug. She calls the clinic and tells you that she missed her last dose. You should tell her:

    a. to double the next dose

    b. not to double the next dose

    c. to take half the dosage with the next dose

    d. to skip the next dose

CHAPTER 40

Antifungal Drugs

■ Exercises

Match the following.

1. ____ saprophytes
2. ____ nystatin (Mycostatin)
3. ____ terbinafine (Lamisil)
4. ____ naftifine (Naftin)
5. ____ griseofulvin (Fulvicin)
6. ____ miconazole (Monistat)
7. ____ dermatophytes
8. ____ amphotericin B (Fungizone)
9. ____ sporotrichosis
10. ____ parasitic
11. ____ histoplasmosis
12. ____ glucan
13. ____ itraconazole (Sporanox)
14. ____ flucytosine (Ancobon)
15. ____ mycoses
16. ____ caspofungin (Cancidas)
17. ____ echinocandins
18. ____ Amphotec
19. ____ aspergillosis
20. ____ oral candidiasis

a. Fungi that obtain food from living organisms
b. Antifungal drug that should be taken with fatty meal
c. Oral antifungal drug used to treat onychomycosis
d. Antifungal drug used to treat serious systemic fungal infections
e. Fungi that obtain food from dead organic matter
f. Occurs when contaminated material seeps through the skin via wounds on the body
g. Popular antifungal agent used to treat vulvovaginal candidiasis
h. Fungi that grow at cooler body surface temperatures
i. Antifungal drug used to treat athlete's foot and jock itch
j. A polyene agent used topically to treat oral, intestinal, or vaginal candidiasis
k. Fungus found in soil and organic matter around chicken houses, bird roosts, and bat caves
l. Component of fungal walls
m. Drug of choice for histoplasmosis
n. Fungal infections
o. Indicated for treatment of invasive aspergillosis in clients who cannot take Amphotericin B or itraconazole
p. Antifungal drugs that disrupt fungal cell walls, rather than fungal cell membranes
q. Mainly used to treat yeast infections
r. Lipid preparation of amphotericin B
s. The most common invasive mold infection
t. Painless, white plaques on oral pharyngeal mucosa

Place T (true) or F (false) in each blank.

1. ____ People may develop histoplasmosis years after the primary infection.

2. ____ Fungi are smaller and less complex than bacteria.

3. ____ Most invasive fungal infections are acquired by inhalation of airborne spores.

4. ____ Drugs for superficial fungal infections are usually taken orally.

5. ____ Amphotericin B is highly toxic to humans.

6. ____ All azoles are contraindicated in pregnancy.

7. ____ Multiple doses of fluconazole (Diflucan) are needed for vaginal candidiasis.

8. ____ Adverse effects are uncommon with caspofungin.

9. ____ Griseofulvin is contraindicated for clients with renal disease.

10. ____ Therapeutic effects of terbinafine (Lamisil) may not be evident for several months after the drug is stopped.

■ Clinical Challenge

Your client is a 72-year-old male who has battled emphysema for many years. He is admitted to the hospital with a possible diagnosis of aspergillosis. He is started on amphotericin B. Which adverse effects will you look for? If the client develops hypertension, edema, or hypokalemia, what should you do?

■ Review Questions

1. Griseofulvin (Fulvicin) has been prescribed for your client who has a fingernail infection. When discussing the drug with her, she states that she is afraid of the adverse effects of the drug, especially an allergic reaction. An appropriate response would be:

    a. "Adverse effects are very common with this drug. We will monitor you very closely for these effects."

    b. "This drug causes very serious adverse effects. You could die!"

    c. "There is a very low incidence of serious reactions to this drug."

    d. "Don't worry about it. You probably won't experience any ill effects from the drug."

2. Your client, age 50, is taking amphotericin B (Fungizone) IV. Which of the following electrolyte imbalances will you look for?

    a. hyperkalemia

    b. hypokalemia

    c. hypernatremia

    d. hyponatremia

3. You are to administer nystatin suspension to your client, who has thrush. Which of the following will you include in your instructions to the client regarding administration?

    a. Swish and swallow.

    b. Hold in mouth for 2 minutes, then spit out.

    c. Swallow immediately.

    d. Use a cotton swab to apply to mouth lesions.

4. Your client has a tinea infection of the scalp. Itraconazole (Sporanox) capsules have been ordered. What will you tell her in regard to taking the capsules?

    a. "Take prior to a meal."

    b. "Take after a full meal."

    c. "Take with a full glass of water."

    d. "Take with just enough water to swallow the capsule."

5. Your client is taking amphotericin B for aspergillosis. Which of the following lab values would indicate that the medication should not be given?

   a. hematocrit of 45%

   b. blood urea nitrogen of 62 mg/dL

   c. bilirubin (total) of 0.8 mg/dL

   d. sodium 142 mEq/L

6. Fluconazole (Diflucan) 400 mg/d PO has been prescribed for a client who has HIV. He should be instructed to notify his health care provider immediately if he experiences:

   a. headaches and slight dizziness

   b. dryness and itching of skin

   c. nausea and constipation

   d. unusual fatigue and dark urine

7. Your client has tinea pedis. Haloprogin (Halo-tex) 1% cream daily has been prescribed. Which of the following instructions should be given to the client?

   a. Wash hair before applying cream to scalp.

   b. Wash and dry feet before applying the cream.

   c. Do not wet area before application of cream.

   d. Apply cream and remove after 30 minutes.

8. Which of the following drugs should not be taken with oral ketoconazole (Nizoral)?

   a. Prilosec

   b. ASA

   c. folic acid

   d. Digoxin

9. Which of the following is the most common and most serious adverse effect of Amphotericin B?

   a. hepatoxicity

   b. cardiotoxicity

   c. nephrotoxicity

   d. ototoxicity

10. Your client has a diagnosis of oral candidiasis. Which of the following drugs do you expect her to be placed on?

    a. nystatin (Mycostatin)

    b. natamycin (Natacyn)

    c. naftifine (Naftin)

    d. ketoconazole (Nizoral)

CHAPTER 41

Antiparasitics

■ Exercises

Match the following.

1. _____ trichomoniasis

2. _____ scabies

3. _____ amebiasis

4. _____ tapeworm

5. _____ roundworm

6. _____ toxoplasmosis

7. _____ pediculosis

8. _____ giardiasis

9. _____ trichinosis

10. _____ pinworm

11. _____ helminthiasis

12. _____ hookworm

13. _____ pneumocystosis

14. _____ threadworm

15. _____ malaria

a. Caused by ingesting undercooked meat or contact with feces from infected cats

b. A parasitic infestation of the skin caused by the itch mite

c. Vaginal infection spread by sexual intercourse

d. A parasitic infestation of the skin caused by lice

e. An acute, life-threatening respiratory infection

f. Produces a potentially serious infection that can enter all body tissue

g. Infestation with parasitic worms

h. The most common parasitic worm infection in the United States

i. Usually transmitted by larvae burrowing through the soles of bare feet

j. Transmitted by *Anopheles* spp. mosquitoes to humans

k. A worm infection caused by ingestion of under-cooked meat, especially pork

l. Most common parasitic worm infection in the world

m. A common disease found in Africa, Asia, and Latin America

n. A helminthic infection that produces proglottids

o. Caused by an intestinal parasite and can be found in people who camp or hike in wilderness areas

■ Clinical Challenge

Your client is going on a medical/construction mission trip to Africa. She is in the clinic for her physical exam and immunization update. The nurse discusses the need for malaria prophylaxis. The physician prescribes chloroquine with primaquine. What will the nurse teach the client regarding these drugs?

■ Review Questions

1. Your client is taking pyrimethamine (Daraprim) for the prevention of malaria. Because this drug interferes with folic acid metabolism, you will observe for:

   a. hypotension

   b. anemia

   c. depression

   d. diabetes mellitus

2. A sexually active 18-year-old female client is taking Flagyl for trichomoniasis. A primary concern for the health care provider would be:

   a. the administration of the drug three times daily for 7 days

   b. the decrease in severity of symptoms

   c. the treatment of the client's sexual partner

   d. the adverse effects of the drug

3. The mother of a 5-year-old boy who is taking pyrantel (Antiminth) for pinworms asks you when she can be sure that the drug has worked. Your best response should be:

   a. "After 6 weeks of therapy, we can assume the pinworms have been eradicated."

   b. "It will take 2 to 3 months after drug therapy to be sure there are no more pinworms."

   c. "One negative stool culture will indicate the pinworms are gone."

   d. "We will need three negative stool cultures before your son is considered free of the worms."

4. You are taking care of a missionary who has spent a year in Asia. He is being treated with iodoquinol (Yodoxin) for intestinal amebiasis. Which of the following statements would you expect from your client?

   a. "I'm not sure where I am."

   b. "I'm experiencing severe headaches."

   c. "I have heartburn."

   d. "I wish this nausea would go away."

5. A 28-year-old male was recently diagnosed with AIDS. He is being treated through a private clinic specializing in immunosuppressed clients. He is taking trimethoprim-sulfamethoxazole (Bactrium) for pneumocystosis. A common adverse effect of this drug is:

   a. skin rash

   b. increased blood pressure

   c. difficulty in swallowing

   d. dizziness

6. When teaching a young mother about treatment of pediculosis capitis for her 5-year-old, the nurse will stress the importance of:

   a. drug therapy, including measures to avoid reinfection or transmission to others

   b. keeping her child from playing in dirt

   c. keeping the child isolated from other children for at least 2 weeks

   d. avoiding raw fish and undercooked meat

7. When instructing a client who has malaria regarding administration of chloroquine (Aralen), the nurse should include:

   a. Take medication with or after meals.

   b. Drink a full glass of water with each dose.

   c. Take 2 hours before meals.

   d. Avoid dairy products when taking the medication.

8. You are discussing the use of permethrin (OTC: Nix) for treatment of head lice with a grandmother of a 6-year-old. Which of the following would be an appropriate statement to her?

   a. "Leave the medication on longer than the directions indicate."

   b. "Decrease the amount of the medication indicated in the directions."

   c. "Leaving the medication on longer than indicated can cause seizures."

   d. "Do not leave the medication on as long as the directions indicate."

9. How does phenobarbital alter the effects of metronidazole (Flagyl)?

   a. It increases the effects by decreasing hepatic metabolism of Flagyl.

   b. It decreases effects of Flagyl by increasing its rate of hepatic metabolism.

   c. It causes a decreased rate of urinary excretion.

   d. It increases the risk of Flagyl toxicity and retinal damage by inhibiting metabolism.

10. Your client is taking quinine for malaria and is complaining of headaches, tinnitus, difficulty hearing, and blurred vision. You suspect that he is experiencing:

    a. vertigo

    b. hypocalcemia

    c. pruritus

    d. cinchonism

CHAPTER 42

Physiology of the Hematopoietic and Immune Systems

■ Exercises

Fill in the blank.

1. _____ regulate blood cell activity by working as chemical messengers.

2. _____ interfere with the ability of viruses to replicate in uninfected cells.

3. _____ facilitate movement of leukocytes into injured tissue.

4. The _____ _____ helps protect the body from harmful substances.

5. The body's main external defense mechanism is _____ _____.

6. _____ is a generalized response to tissue damage that helps in tissue repair.

7. The attraction of white blood cells to injured tissue areas is called _____.

8. _____ _____ markers regulate antigens and allow immune cells to communicate with each other.

9. _____ _____ is when antibodies are formed by the immune system of another person or animal and is transferred to the host.

10. Foreign substances that initiate immune responses are called _____.

11. _____ are proteins that interact with specific antigens.

12. _____ cells are white blood cells found throughout the body in lymphoid tissues.

13. _____ contain inflammatory mediators or digestive enzymes.

14. _____ are the body's main defense against pathogenic bacteria.

15. In parasitic infections, _____ bind to and kill parasites.

16. _____ release histamine.

17. _____ _____ are the main regulators of immune responses.

18. In _____ disorders, the body perceives its own tissues as antigens and causes an immune response.

19. In _____ disorders, the body perceives normally harmless substances as antigens and produces an immune response.

20. _____ immunity involves B lymphocytes and antibodies in the blood.

■ Review Questions

1. The main function of interferons is to:
   a. stimulate growth of bone marrow
   b. inhibit viral replication in uninfected cells
   c. promote growth of monocyte-macrophages
   d. activate growth of T cells

2. Hematopoietic agents are used to prevent or treat:

   a. symptoms of diseases and/or adverse side effects of their treatments

   b. neoplastic diseases

   c. allergic disorders

   d. adverse effects of drugs used to replace iron in the body

3. The process in which weak extracts of antigenic substances are prepared as a drug and administered in small, increasing amounts to develop a tolerance for the substance iscalled:

   a. immunosuppression

   b. detoxification

   c. activation

   d. desensitization

4. An inadequate amount of which of the following minerals can depress the functions of T and B cells?

   a. magnesium

   b. iron

   c. zinc

   d. copper

5. The mother of a 14-day-old baby girl is concerned that the baby has been exposed to chickenpox. An appropriate response to her would be:

   a. "Let your pediatrician know as soon as you notice a rash on the baby."

   b. "The baby should be covered by maternal antibodies until approximately 6 months of age."

   c. "Don't worry, the baby will be okay."

   d. "The baby's immune system is still immature. She will probably contract the virus."

6. B lymphocytes that are capable of forming antibodies originate in:

   a. stem cells in bone marrow

   b. lymph nodes

   c. neutrophils

   d. antigens

7. Which of the following immunoglobulins is stimulated in anaphylaxis?

   a. IgA

   b. IgM

   c. IgE

   d. IgG

8. Which of the following is *not* a method of target cell destruction by T cells?

   a. formation of holes in the target cells that allow fluids to enter and cause the cell to swell and burst

   b. activation of specific antigens as chemical messengers to break down cell components

   c. insertion of enzymes that break down or digest the cell

   d. initiation of programmed cell death (apoptosis)

9. Which of the following lymphocytes do not need to interact with a specific antigen to become activated?

   a. R cells

   b. T cells

   c. B cells

   d. natural killer cells

10. Which of the following *best* describes acquired immunity?

    a. Antibodies are formed by the immune system of another person or animal and transferred to the host.

    b. It is a general, protective mechanism activated by major histocompatibility complex.

    c. It is produced by a person's own immune system in response to a disease caused by a specific antigen from a source outside the body.

    d. Antibodies or B cells come in contact with antigens in the blood or other body fluids.

CHAPTER 43

Immunizing Agents

■ Exercises

Place a T (true) or F (false) in each blank.

1. ____ Antigens that activate the immune response can be microorganisms that cause infectious diseases.

2. ____ It is recommended that only activated polio vaccine be used in the United States.

3. ____ Hepatitis B virus (HBV) infection can cause liver disease.

4. ____ HBV is recommended for at-risk people only.

5. ____ Immunization against diphtheria and tetanus is one time only for life.

6. ____ Vaccines should *not* be given together.

7. ____ Immunization involves administration of an antibody to produce an antigen.

8. ____ Attenuated vaccines are weakened or reduced in virulence, which can cause mild forms of the disease.

9. ____ Most often, attenuated live vaccines produce lifelong immunity.

10. ____ Toxoids are chemical toxins that have been changed to destroy toxicity yet still are able to initiate antibody formation.

11. ____ Toxoid immunity is *not* permanent, and repeated doses are needed.

12. ____ Vaccines containing aluminum should be given by mouth.

13. ____ Vaccines and toxoids should not be given during febrile illnesses.

14. ____ The best source for information concerning current recommendations is the Centers for Disease Control and Prevention (CDC).

15. ____ The measles-mumps-rubella (MMR) vaccine should be stored away from light.

16. ____ Most vaccines require refrigeration.

17. ____ MMR is given to infants at 6 months of age.

18. ____ Pneumococcal vaccine is *not* recommended for children.

19. ____ Varicella vaccine should be given twice by 12 years of age.

20. ____ Health care workers should have a tetanus-diphtheria booster every 10 years.

21. ____ High-risk groups and health care providers should receive the influenza vaccine annually.

22. ____ A booster may be needed following the hepatitis B vaccine.

23. ____ Live vaccines should *not* be given to people with cancer.

24. ____ Children with HIV infection should receive all immunizations.

25. ____ *Haemophilus influenzae* type b (Hib) conjugate vaccine is given to prevent serious bacterial infections, including meningitis.

■ Clinical Challenge

A mother of a pre-college student calls the clinic and is clearly upset. She explains that her son is being denied admission to the college of his choice because he does not have an immunization record. After asking her a few questions, you determine that her husband is in the military and that they have lived in seven states over the past 15 years. She tells you that she is sure that her son received all vaccines, but she can't find the immunization card. What do you tell her? What would you tell a new mother concerning recordkeeping of immunizations?

■ Review Questions

1. A mother has brought her 15-month-old daughter to the health department for diphtheria-tetanus-pertussis (DTaP) and MMR vaccines. Which of the following drugs should be suggested for fever and soreness at the injection site?

   a. Aspirin

   b. Advil

   c. Tylenol

   d. Motrin

2. A 20-year-old female is given a rubella immunization. Which of the following statements by the nurse is *most* important?

   a. "You may take Tylenol for the fever and pain.'

   b. "You must use effective birth control for at least 3 months."

   c. "You may experience flu-like symptoms."

   d. "You should take it easy for about 3 days."

3. A young mother has brought her 6-month-old baby into the clinic for immunizations. The nurse should assess for:

   a. fever

   b. weight loss

   c. anemia

   d. slowed development

4. After a baby receives a DTaP the nurse will teach the mother to watch for which of the following potential adverse effects?

   a. anorexia and nausea

   b. tremors and possible seizures

   c. difficulty swallowing and abdominal distention

   d. diarrhea and abdominal pain

5. Which of the following drugs decrease the overall effects of vaccines?

   a. acetaminophen (Tylenol)

   b. diazepam (Valium)

   c. furosemide (Lasix)

   d. phenytoin (Dilantin)

6. In assessing immunization needs of your client who will be leaving for Asia in several weeks, you explain that he should receive a tetanus toxoid injection if he has not had one in the last:

   a. 6 months

   b. year

   c. 5 years

   d. 10 years

7. The hepatitis B vaccine is recommended as early as:

   a. a few hours after birth

   b. 6 months of age

   c. 1 year of age

   d. 6 years of age

8. You must give RhoGAM to your Rh-negative client who just delivered an Rh-positive baby within:

   a. 1 hour

   b. 6 hours

   c. 24 hours

   d. 72 hours

9. You have just administered vaccines to three children. You explained to their mother that she must wait with the children in the clinic for at least:

a. 15 minutes

b. 30 minutes

c. 1 hour

d. 1½ hours

10. Which of the following drugs should be readily available when administering any immunization?

a. Tylenol

b. Valium

c. Epinephrine

d. Lasix

CHAPTER 44

Hematopoietic and Immunostimulant Drugs

■Exercises

Answer the following.

1. Why are hematopoietic and immunostimulant drugs given?

2. What are the disadvantages of using cytokines?

3. How do interferons weaken viruses?

4. How does bacillus Calmette-Guérin (BCG) vaccine act against cancer of the urinary bladder?

5. Why are hematopoietic and immunostimulant drugs given subcutaneously or intravenously?

Fill in the blank.

1. _____ is used to prevent severe thrombocytopenia and reduces the need for platelet transfusions in clients with cancer who are taking chemotherapy.

2. _____ are used to treat viral infections and cancers.

3. _____ _____ and _____ are used to treat or prevent anemia.

4. _____ is used to treat metastatic renal cell carcinoma and melanoma.

5. _____ helps prevent infection by decreasing the incidence, severity, and duration of neutropenia associated with chemotherapy.

6. _____ _____ ____ _____ is used to treat adults with genital warts.

7. _____ is an interferon beta-1a used to treat multiple sclerosis.

8. _____ agents increase the effects of interferons.

9. _____ decrease the effects of aldesleukin.

10. Acute, flu-like symptoms are more likely to occur with _____.

▪ Clinical Challenge

A client is taking interferon alfa-2a for hairy cell leukemia. He has been discharged from the hospital. A caregiver will administer the injections. Why is it important that the medication be administered as prescribed? What would the nurse stress to the caregiver concerning this medication?

▪ Review Questions

1. The nurse should be aware that immunostimulant therapy:
   a. should be administered by mouth
   b. involves shaking the medication vigorously before preparing the administration
   c. has very few and minor adverse effects
   d. can cause anaphylactic or other allergic reactions to occur

2. Your client is receiving darbepoetin alfa (Aranesp) for anemia associated with chronic renal failure. You will omit a dose if the hemoglobin level is:
   a. >2 g/dL
   b. >5 g/dL
   c. >8 g/dL
   d. >12 g/dL

3. A client is being treated with aldesleukin (Proleukin) for metastatic renal cell carcinoma. He has just experienced a severe reaction from the medication. You suspect that his physician will:
   a. decrease the dosage of the drug
   b. withhold one or more doses
   c. add a second drug to decrease adverse effect
   d. continue with prescribed dosage and see whether reaction occurs again

4. Which of the following should be monitored before and during treatment with darbepoetin alfa and epoetin alfa?
   a. transferrin saturation and serum ferritin
   b. serum amylase and nucleotidase
   c. thrombin clotting time and prothrombin time
   d. complete blood count and platelet count

5. Your client has neutropenia as a result of chemotherapy. In order to prevent infection, filgrastim (Neupogen) will be started:
   a. immediately after the last dose of chemotherapy
   b. 24 hours after the last dose of chemotherapy
   c. in between chemotherapy doses
   d. 2 weeks after chemotherapy has ended

6. Aldesleukin is contraindicated in clients with preexisting:
   a. diabetes mellitus
   b. Parkinson's disease
   c. spastic colon or diverticulitis
   d. cardiovascular or pulmonary disease

7. Oprelvekin (Neumega) is being given to your 7-year-old client who has thrombocytopenia. You will observe for which of the following adverse effects?
   a. hypertension
   b. bradycardia
   c. tachycardia
   d. hypotension

8. You are aware that your client had a preexisting renal impairment before she started sargramostim therapy. You will monitor which of the following?
   a. serum creatinine levels
   b. electrolyte levels
   c. blood glucose levels
   d. aspartate transaminase levels

9. Your 78-year-old client is taking oprelvekin (Neumega). Which of the following adverse effects is most likely to occur in your client?

    a. bone pain

    b. atrial dysrrhythmias

    c. increased uric acid

    d. arthralgias levels

10. A favorable outcome for a client who is on epoetin alfa therapy would be:

    a. increase in hematocrit

    b. decrease in hemoglobin

    c. increase in white blood cells

    d. decrease in red blood cells

CHAPTER 45

Immunosuppressants

▪ Exercises

Match the following.

1. _____ azathioprine (Imuran)

2. _____ mycophenolate mefetil (CellCept)

3. _____ lymphocyte immune globulin (Atgam)

4. _____ infliximab (Remicade)

5. _____ corticosteroids

6. _____ etanercept (Enbrel)

7. _____ tacrolimus (Prograf)

8. _____ cyclosporine (Sandimmune)

9. _____ methotrexate (Rheumatrex)

10. _____ antiproliferative agents

a. A folate antagonist that inhibits production and function of immune cells

b. Insoluble in water, formulated in alcohol, olive oil, and castor oil

c. Antimetabolite that interferes with production of RNA and DNA

d. Obtained from the serum of horses immunized with human thymus tissue or lymphocytes

e. A monoclonal antibody used to treat rheumatoid arthritis and Crohn's disease

f. Group of drugs used therapeutically as immuno-suppressants

g. Less toxic than azathioprine and has synergistic effects with corticosteroids

h. A tumor necrosis factor receptor used to treat rheumatoid arthritis when other treatments have failed

i. Drugs that damage or kill cells that are able to reproduce

j. Children require higher doses to maintain plasma drug levels

Place a T (true) or F (false) in each blank.

1. _____ The immune response is an important factor in the success or failure of an organ transplant.

2. _____ In autoimmune disorders, a person's body can differentiate between self-antigens and foreign antigens.

3. _____ Most autoantigens are protein in nature.

4. _____ In organ and tissue transplantation, the goal is to rid the body of immunosuppression.

5. _____ Immunosuppression can cause serious infections in the body.

6. _____ A rejection reaction occurs when the host's immune system is activated to destroy the transplanted organ.

7. _____ In a rejection reaction, the initial target of the recipient antibodies is the blood vessels surrounding the transplanted organ.

8. _____ Chronic rejection reactions cause a gradual decrease in serum creatinine levels.

9. _____ Chronic graft-versus-host disease occurs when symptoms last or occur 1 month after transplantation.

10. _____ Long-term use of immunosuppressant drugs can cause cancer.

■ Clinical Challenge

An 81-year-old male has a diagnosis of severe rheumatoid arthritis and has had a progressive treatment regimen of prednisone, methotrexate, infliximab (Remicade), and leflunomide (Arava). During a clinical treatment of Remicade, he and his wife voice concern about adverse effects of all the medication he is taking. How should the nurse respond?

■ Review Questions

1. Clients on long-term immunosuppressant drug therapy with autoimmune disorders and organ transplantation are at increased risk for:

   a. hypotension

   b. osteoporosis

   c. cancer

   d. chronic urinary tract infections

2. Before a client is put on cyclosporine (Sandimmune) to help prevent a rejection reaction from a liver transplant, the nurse should assess for which of the following?

   a. use of alcohol

   b. weight loss

   c. blood glucose level

   d. activity level

3. Your client has had a heart transplant and is receiving cyclosporine (Sandimmune) as part of his postoperative treatment plan. A major adverse effect of this drug is:

   a. hepatotoxicity

   b. hypersensitive reactions

   c. nephrotoxicity

   d. nausea and vomiting

4. Sirolimus (Rapamune) is given in combination with cyclosporine (Sandimmune) to prevent renal transplant rejection. The two drugs given 4 hours apart have a greater total effect than the sum of their individual effects. This drug action is:

   a. synergism

   b. simple summation

   c. potentiation

   d. antagonism

5. Your client is receiving an antibody preparation, lymphocyte immune globulin (Atgam). You will administer the medication:

   a. by mouth

   b. by the intradermal method

   c. subcutaneously

   d. intravenously

6. You work in a rheumatology clinic where infliximab (Remicade) is administered. Which of the following drugs should be available for easy access if necessary?

   a. B_{12}

   b. Dramamine

   c. Maalox

   d. Epinephrine

7. Your client is taking azathioprine (Imuran) to prevent renal transplant rejection. In order to assess for bone marrow depression which of the following lab results should be monitored?

   a. white blood cell and platelet counts

   b. red blood cell and platelet counts

   c. complete blood cell and platelet counts

   d. white blood cell and plasma counts

8. Which of the following elevated lab results could indicate hepatotoxicity from the use of cyclosporine (Sandimmune)?

   a. serum aminotransferases and bilirubin

   b. blood glucose level and ketone count

   c. urine specify gravity and urine pH

   d. arterial blood gases and O_2 saturation

9. Your client has been placed on methotrexate (Rheumatrex) therapy for rheumatoid arthritis. You will monitor the client throughout therapy for:

a. peripheral neuropathy

b. hyperthyroidism

c. nephrotoxicity

d. hepatotoxicity

10. You are preparing an oral dose of cyclosporine (Sandimmune) for your client. You will mix the medication with:

a. room-temperature apple juice

b. cold orange juice

c. lukewarm grapefruit juice

d. cold milk

CHAPTER 46

Physiology of the Respiratory System

■ Exercises

Match the following.

1. _____ diffusion

2. _____ ventilation

3. _____ cilia

4. _____ compliance

5. _____ lobule

6. _____ respiration

7. _____ nasopharynx

8. _____ pleura

9. _____ alveoli

10. _____ perfusion

a. Process of gas exchange by which oxygen is obtained and carbon dioxide is eliminated

b. Tiny hair-like projections that move mucous toward the pharynx to be expectorated or swallowed

c. Grape-like cluster of air sacs

d. Functions as a passageway and air "conditioner" that helps warm, humidify, and filter incoming air

e. The process by which oxygen and carbon dioxide are transferred between alveoli and blood, and between blood and body cells

f. Ability of lungs to stretch or expand to accommodate incoming air

g. Membranes that encase the lungs

h. The movement of air between the atmosphere and the alveoli of the lungs

i. Blood flow through the lungs

j. Functional unit of the lung where gas exchange takes place

Answer the following.

1. What percentage of oxygen is in atmospheric air?

2. How many times per minute does normal breathing occur?

3. How much air is inspired and expired with a normal breath?

4. How many times an hour do deep breaths or sighs occur?

5. List common signs and symptoms of respiratory disorders.

■ Review Questions

1. Permanent brain damage from lack of oxygen occurs within:
   a. 1 to 2 minutes
   b. 4 to 6 minutes
   c. 10 to 15 minutes
   d. 20 to 30 minutes

2. Carbon dioxide is considered a:
   a. necessary component of cell metabolism
   b. nontoxic gas
   c. major waste product of cell metabolism
   d. liquid

3. Which of the following is not part of the respiratory tract?
   a. Henle's loop
   b. nose
   c. pharynx
   d. bronchi

4. Which of the following is considered an alternate airway?
   a. epiglottis
   b. cochlear
   c. Purkinje fibers
   d. mouth

5. Pharyngeal walls are composed of:
   a. smooth muscle
   b. skeletal muscle
   c. vocal cord
   d. bronchi

6. Which of the following is the passageway between the larynx and main stem bronchi?
   a. pharynx
   b. bronchioles
   c. trachea
   d. nose

7. Which of the following helps protect and defend the lungs?
   a. bronchi and bronchioles
   b. oxygen and carbon dioxide
   c. larynx and pharynx
   d. cilia and mucus

8. Blood enters the lungs through which of the following?
   a. pulmonary artery
   b. pulmonary vein
   c. aorta
   d. coronary arteries

9. Which of the following is a lipoprotein substance that decreases surface tension in the alveoli?
   a. glycerin
   b. surfactant
   c. bile
   d. interferon

10. Which of the following transports oxygen to body cells?
    a. alveoli
    b. B lymphocytes
    c. neutrophils
    d. hemoglobin

■Respiratory System Diagram

Match the letter of the descriptive statement with the corresponding body part in Figure 46-1.

A. Warms and humidifies the air.

B. Where air exchange takes place.

C. Connects the upper and lower respiratory tract.

D. The vocal cords are located here.

E. The walls contain smooth muscle controlled by the autonomic nervous system.

F. This muscle aids in respiration.

G. Mainstem bronchus.

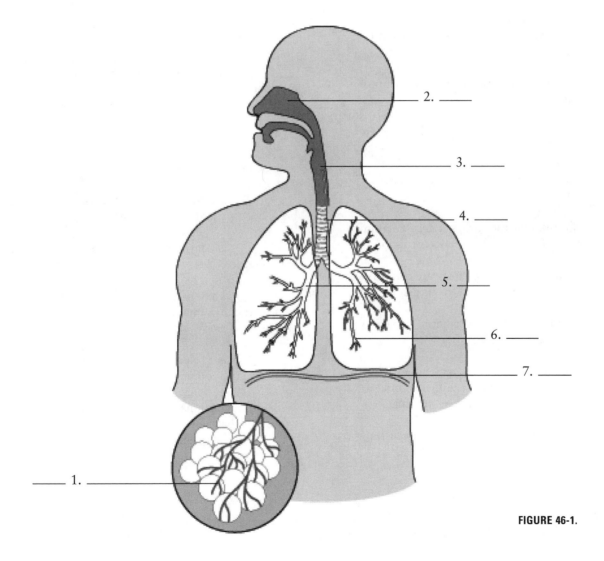

FIGURE 46-1.

CHAPTER 47

Drugs for Asthma and Other Bronchoconstrictive Disorders

■ Exercises

Place a T (true) or F (false) in each blank.

1. ____ Hispanics have a higher death rate from asthma than do other ethnic groups.

2. ____ Children who are exposed to tobacco smoke are at risk for the development of asthma.

3. ____ A chronic cough can be the only symptom of asthma.

4. ____ Asthma is a respiratory disorder characterized by bronchodilation.

5. ____ Anti-asthmatic medications can increase acid reflux.

6. ____ Anti-inflammatory drugs reduce inflammation by increasing bronchoconstriction.

7. ____ Adrenergic bronchodilators are contraindicated in clients with severe cardiac disease.

8. ____ Epinephrine is the treatment of choice to relieve acute asthma.

9. ____ IV administration of a corticosteroid in acute severe asthma has a therapeutic advantage over oral administration.

10. ____ Leukotriene modifiers and mast cell stabilizers cause serious adverse effects.

Fill in the blank.

1. _____ and _____ are used only for prophylaxis of acute bronchoconstriction.

2. _____ is used to prevent exercise-induced asthma.

3. Muscle tremor is the most frequent adverse effect of _____.

4. _____, an anticholinergic agent, is available in a nasal spray to treat rhinorrhea associated with allergic rhinitis and the common cold.

5. _____ therapy is contraindicated in clients with acute gastritis and peptic ulcer disease.

6. _____ are chemical mediators of bronchoconstriction and inflammation.

7. _____ is contraindicated in clients with liver disease.

8. _____, an antichlolinergic bronchodilator, is most effective in long-term management of chronic obstructive pulmonary disease.

9. _____ is a selective beta-2 adrenergic agonist that is a long-acting bronchodilator.

10. With chronic asthma, a _____ is usually taken by inhalation on a daily basis.

■ Clinical Challenge

Your client is a 15-year-old girl who has asthma. She has a short-acting bronchodilator inhaler albuterol (Proventil); however, she states that it "doesn't seem to help." How do you respond?

You determine she is not using the inhaler correctly. What do you do?

You notice that she has difficulty in manually holding and operating the inhaler. What do you recommend?

■ Review Questions

1. A 16-year-old enters the hospital emergency room with a severe asthma attack. Which of the following drugs will most likely be used?

   a. salmeterol

   b. epinephrine

   c. albuterol

   d. formoterol

2. Your asthmatic client's medication has been changed to theophylline (Theo-Dur). Which of the following is most important to include in his client teaching?

   a. Take only on an empty stomach.

   b. Increase intake of fatty foods.

   c. Decrease intake of fluids.

   d. Limit intake of caffeine.

3. When teaching an asthma client the proper technique for administering a metered-dose inhaler, the nurse will emphasize:

   a. not to eat or drink prior to or after administration

   b. to lie in semi-Fowler's position while administering the inhaler

   c. to hold his breath for 10 seconds after inhaling the medication before exhaling

   d. to place his lips firmly around the inhaler's mouthpiece

4. Your client has been diagnosed with asthma. You have just finished explaining the use of a metered-dose inhaler. Which of the following responses indicates the need for further instruction?

   a. "I should inhale deeply before depressing the inhaler."

   b. "I will shake the inhaler well before each use."

   c. "I will wait about 5 minutes before I inhale for the second time."

   d. "I will not use more than one or two puffs per treatment."

5. Your client has been using a beclomethasone (Beclovent) inhaler for several months. She is in the clinic complaining of a rash in her mouth. She is upset and states she knows it is from the inhaler she is using. Which of the following should you do?

   a. Recommend that she stop using the Beclovent inhaler immediately.

   b. Instruct your client to decrease the dosage of Beclovent.

   c. Inform her that she is having an allergic reaction to something she has eaten.

   d. Remind her that she must rinse her mouth after each treatment.

6. Your client has been taking zafirlukast (Accolate) for asthma for 3 weeks. She is in the clinic for a follow-up visit. Which of the following findings would cause you alarm?

   a. pulse rate of 84

   b. absence of wheezing

   c. pink nail beds

   d. whites of eyes are yellow in color

7. A client who is on theophylline (Theo-Dur) is in the clinic for a theophylline level. You know that the optimal therapeutic range for this drug is:

   a. 0.5 to 3 mcg/mL

   b. 5 to 15 mcg/mL

   c. 20 to 30 mcg/mL

   d. 50 to 65 mcg/mL

8. Which of the following drugs is used only for prophylaxis of bronchoconstriction?

   a. epinephrine

   b. salmeterol

   c. isoproterenol

   d. albuterol

9. Your client is taking a combination of ipratropium and albuterol (Combivent). Which of the following will you stress as a common adverse effect?

   a. increased pulse rate

   b. rhinorrhea

   c. weight gain

   d. cough

10. You are instructing your client on the administration of zafirlukast (Accolate). Which of the following should you include in your instructions?

    a. Take 1 hour before or 2 hours after a meal.

    b. Take with fatty foods.

    c. Take medication once daily.

    d. May be taken with or without food.

CHAPTER 48

Antihistamines and Allergic Disorders

■ Exercises

Answer the following.

1. Where is histamine mainly located in the body?

2. What causes histamine to be discharged from mast cells and basophils?

3. Where are H_1 receptors located?

4. List six responses that may occur when histamine binds with H_1 receptors.

5. List three responses that occur when H_2 receptors are stimulated.

Match the following

1. _____ type I allergic reaction

2. _____ urticaria

3. _____ epinephrine

4. _____ anaphylaxis

5. _____ hydroxyzine (Atarax)

6. _____ serum sickness

7. _____ allergic rhinitis

8. _____ antigens

9. _____ anaphylactoid reactions

10. _____ type II allergic reaction

a. Mediated by IgG and IgM

b. Drug of choice for treating severe anaphylaxis

c. A vascular reaction of the skin characterized by papules or wheals and severe itching

d. Example of type I allergic reaction

e. Foreign materials

f. Prescribed for pruritus

g. A delayed hypersensitivity reaction most often caused by drugs

h. Inflammation of nasal mucosa

i. May occur on first exposure to a foreign substance

j. Mediated by IgE

■ Clinical Challenge

Your client, a 65-year-old female, has been prescribed cetirizine (Zyrtec) to treat her seasonal allergies. What assessment data do you need in order to provide client education concerning use of an antihistamine?

■ Review Questions

1. A 25-year-old female calls the clinic at 3:00 PM and tells you she forgot to take her morning dose of fexofenadine (Allegra). She wants to know what she should do. You tell her to:

   a. double her evening dose

   b. skip the evening dose and start back in the morning

   c. forget about the morning dose and take the evening dose early

   d. take the morning dose now and the evening dose at the scheduled time

2. Your client has just been placed on an antihistamine for allergic rhinitis. Which of the following will you be sure to include in your teaching plan regarding antihistamines?

   a. Use sunscreen outdoors.

   b. Weigh daily and note any change in weight.

   c. Reduce fat intake in diet.

   d. Reduce intake of citrus juices.

3. A 32-year-old businessman is in the clinic for allergies. He has to make a major presentation in 3 days, and his allergies are worse. He asks whether the doctor can prescribe another antihistamine for him to use with the loratadine (Claritin) he is already taking. Your best response to him would be:

   a. "Sure, I'll ask right now."

   b. "If you take another antihistamine, you will have to decrease the Claritin dosage."

   c. "You should not take two antihistamines at the same time because of possible severe adverse effects."

   d. "Why do you think you need more medication?"

4. A 22-year-old male is in the clinic for seasonal allergies. He states that he works in construction and operates heavy equipment. Which of the following drugs will be prescribed for him?

   a. desloratadine (Clarinex)

   b. clemastine (Tavist)

   c. promethazine (Phenergan)

   d. chlorpheniramine (Chlor-Trimeton)

5. Antihistamines may be contraindicated for people with:

   a. diabetes mellitus

   b. urinary retention

   c. Alzheimer's disease

   d. multiple sclerosis

6. Your client is taking diphenhydramine (Benadryl) for allergic rhinitis. Which of the following nursing diagnoses would be appropriate, especially during the first few days of therapy?

   a. deficient knowledge: safe and accurate drug use

   b. risk for injury related to drowsiness

   c. deficient knowledge: strategies for minimizing exposure to allergens

   d. risk for activity intolerance related to antihistamine

7. On a return visit to the clinic, your client, a 69-year-old male, complains of difficulty voiding. He was seen 1 week ago for pruritus. You suspect he may have:

   a. prostatic hypertrophy

   b. renal failure

   c. diabetes mellitus

   d. cardiac dysrhythmias

8. Which of the following antihistamines is not recommended for children with chickenpox or flu-like infections?

   a. hydroxyzine (Atarax)

   b. clemastine (Tavist)

   c. chlorpheniramine (Chlor-Trimeton)

   d. diphenhydramine (Benadryl)

9. Your client is to begin taking loratadine (Claritin). She asks you how long will it take to help her allergies. Your response should be:

   a. "You should feel better immediately."

   b. "You should see some effects within 1 to 3 hours of your first dose."

   c. "It will take about 3 weeks before you will see any effects."

   d. "In about 2 days, you should feel better."

10. When instructing your client in taking loratadine (Claritin), you should include which of the following?

    a. Take on an empty stomach.

    b. Chew the tablet and follow with a glass of water.

    c. Take with meals.

    d. Take three times a day.

CHAPTER 49

Nasal Decongestants, Antitussives, and Cold Remedies

■ Exercises

Fill in the blank.

1. The major mode for transmission of the common cold is contamination of _____ or _____ _____.

2. School children may have as many as _____ colds a year.

3. Most often, the common cold is caused by the _____.

4. Once a cold virus enters the body, the incubation period is about _____ days.

5. _____ _____ is the most important protective and preventive measure for the common cold.

6. _____ and upper respiratory tract infections are the most common causes of sinusitis.

7. In the central nervous system, the cough center is located in the _____ _____.

8. _____ is secretions discharged from the nose.

9. _____ are administered by inhalation to liquefy mucus in the respiratory tract.

10. The common cold is a _____ infection of the upper respiratory tract.

Designate ingredients for drugs listed below by placing a check mark in the appropriate boxes.

Drug	Antihistamine	Nasal decongestant	Analgesic	Antitussive	Expectorant
Sinutab, sinus, allergy					
TheraFlu, flu, cold, cough					
NyQuil, cold, flu					
Contact, day, night, cold, flu					
Advil, cold, sinus					
Actifed, cold, allergy					
Cheracol D, cough, liquid					
Comtrex, cold, sinus					
Coricidin D, cold					

■ Clinical Challenge

A 70-year-old female was in the clinic 1 week ago complaining of watery eyes, stuffy nose, scratchy throat, and fatigue. It was determined that she had a viral infection and was given pseudoephedrine (Sudafed). Today she is complaining of a headache and dizziness, and she states that she feels worse than she did a week ago. What assessment information does the nurse need to obtain?

Assessment findings are all negative. Due to the client's age and the medication she was given on her initial visit, what do you suspect?

■ Review Questions

1. Your client is a 74-year-old female who is taking pseudoephedrine (Sudafed) for nasal congestion. Which of the following adverse effects will you monitor her for?

   a. increased blood pressure

   b. diarrhea

   c. irritability

   d. constipation

2. Which of the following instructions would the nurse give to a client who is taking an antitussive with codeine?

   a. Avoid coffee, tea, and caffeine drinks.

   b. Decrease fluid intake.

   c. Increase protein in diet.

   d. Avoid alcohol.

3. Which of the following instructions will you give to your client who is taking pseudoephedrine (Dimetapp) in order to facilitate the therapeutic effect of the drug?

   a. Increase fluid intake.

   b. Decrease sodium in diet.

   c. Decrease physical activity.

   d. Take with a glass of milk.

4. A 32-year-old male is in the clinic complaining of a chronic, nonproductive cough. Which of the following drugs will be prescribed for him?

   a. guaifenesin (Robitussin)

   b. dextromethorphan (Benylin DM)

   c. acetylcysteine (Mucomyst)

   d. naphazoline (Privine)

5. You are instructing a 12-year-old boy on how to self-administer a nasal spray. Which of the following will be your initial instruction to him?

   a. "Sit with your neck hyperextended."

   b. "Squeeze the container twice before you spray in each nostril."

   c. "Blow your nose gently."

   d. "Cough up as much mucus as you can."

6. You are instructing a mother on how to administer cough syrup to her 8-year-old. You will include which of the following?

   a. Avoid eating or drinking 30 minutes after administration.

   b. Do not eat or drink 15 minutes prior to administration.

   c. Have the child lie down for 10 minutes after each dose.

   d. Avoid hot baths after taking the medication.

7. A middle-aged woman calls the clinic and states that she has a cold and that she has been using an over-the-counter (OTC) cold remedy for 3 days. She asks you whether she should continue. An appropriate response would be:

   a. "No, you should come into the clinic for prescription medication."

   b. "If you are not better in 1 week, you should come to the clinic."

   c. "You should be okay in a couple of days."

   d. "Yes, you can take OTC medication up to 14 days."

8. Your client, who has been diagnosed with congestive heart failure, is in the clinic for a cold. The physician orders a topical nasal decongestant. Oral agents are contraindicated in this client because these drugs:

a. increase heart rate and blood pressure

b. increase heart rate and decrease blood pressure

c. decrease heart rate and blood pressure

d. decrease heart rate and increase blood pressure

9. Acetylcysteine, a mucolytic, produces a therapeutic effect within:

a. 1 minute

b. 3 minutes

c. 5 minutes

d. 10 minutes

10. An adverse effect of overuse of nasal sprays is:

a. sweaty palms

b. rebound nasal congestion

c. nosebleeds

d. diarrhea

CHAPTER 50

Physiology of the Cardiovascular System

■ Exercises

Answer the following.

1. List two general functions of the cardiovascular system.

2. Describe the heart.

3. What is the main function of the heart valves?

4. Define collateral circulation.

5. Describe the function of capillaries.

Match the following.

1. ____ blood

2. ____ left ventricle

3. ____ endocardium

4. ____ right ventricle

5. ____ myocardium

6. ____ right atrium

7. ____ SA node

8. ____ capacitance

9. ____ pericardium

10. ____ left atrium

a. Receives oxygenated blood from the lungs
b. Fibroserous sac that encloses the heart
c. Functions to nourish and oxygenate body cells
d. Receives deoxygenated blood from superior and inferior vena cava
e. The normal pacemaker of the heart
f. Sends deoxygenated blood through the pulmonary circulation
g. Contracts against high pressure to pump oxygenated blood through the body
h. Membrane lining the heart chambers
i. Veins and venules that assist blood flow against gravity
j. Muscular layer of the heart that provides the pumping action for blood circulation

■ Review Questions

1. Which of the following structures separates the right and left sides of the heart?
   a. mitral valve
   b. epicardium
   c. septum
   d. ventricles

2. If a client had a conduction malformation in his heart, the nurse would suspect a problem with the:

   a. endocardium

   b. SA node

   c. collateral circulation

   d. aortic valve

3. Through the release of epinephrine and norepinephrine, sympathetic nerves:

   a. increase heart rate

   b. decrease heart rate

   c. cause the myocardium to stop contracting

   d. cause collateral circulation

4. Which of the following vessels drain tissue fluid that has filtered through capillaries?

   a. arteries

   b. lymphatic

   c. veins

   d. venules

5. Platelets are necessary for:

   a. defense against microorganisms

   b. blood coagulation

   c. blood cell replication

   d. oxygen transportation

6. Most leukocytes are produced in the:

   a. bone marrow

   b. spleen

   c. liver

   d. lymph nodes

7. What percentage of the total blood volume is plasma?

   a. 10%

   b. 25%

   c. 55%

   d. 85%

8. The primary function of erythrocytes is to:

   a. decrease peripheral vascular resistance

   b. alter the heart rhythm

   c. restore homeostasis

   d. transport oxygen

9. Which of the following valves separate the left atrium and left ventricle?

   a. mitral

   b. tricuspid

   c. pulmonic

   d. aortic

10. Which of the following blood cells produce antibodies?

    a. erythrocytes

    b. leukocytes

    c. platelets

    d. fribrinogen

■ Cardiovascular Diagram

Fill in the blanks in Figure 50-1 with the terms below.

Aorta	Papillary muscle
Right atrium	Left atrium
Mitral valve	Superior vena cava
Coronary arteries	Septum
Pulmonary artery	Left ventricle
Right ventricle	Inferior vena cava
Tricuspid valve	Chordae tendon

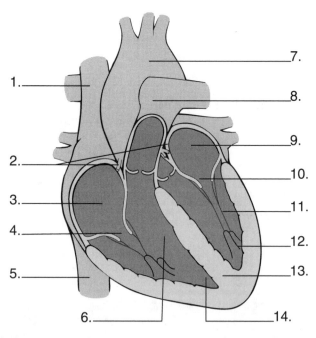

FIGURE 50-1.

CHAPTER 51

Drug Therapy of Heart Failure

■ Exercises

Define the following.

1. Heart failure

2. Endothelin

3. Digitalization

Answer the following.

1. What are the most common conditions leading to heart failure?

2. Explain how the release of renin into the bloodstream can cause heart failure.

Place T (true) or F (false) in each blank.

1. ____ Clients with compensated heart failure exhibit dyspnea and fatigue at rest.

2. ____ Digoxin toxicity may occur at any serum level.

3. ____ Digoxin is the drug of choice for clients with acute myocardial infarction.

4. ____ The onset of action for oral digoxin is 30 minutes to 2 hours.

5. ____ Maximum drug effects of digoxin occur in about 1 week.

6. ____ The drug of choice for acute heart failure is an angiotensin-converting enzyme (ACE) inhibitor.

7. ____ In chronic heart failure, there is a high risk for hypokalemia.

8. ____ Digoxin dosage must be reduced by approximately half in clients with renal failure.

9. ____ In the management of digoxin toxicity, potassium chloride may be given if the serum potassium level is low.

10 ____ In children, there is a significant difference between a therapeutic dose and a toxic dose.

11. ____ Digoxin toxicity develops more often and lasts longer in renal impairment.

12. ____ Hepatic impairment has a tremendous effect on digoxin clearance, and dosage adjustments must be made.

13. ____ Ephedra may be used by clients with heart failure.

14. ____ A client may substitute the brand and type of digoxin.

15. ____ In atrial fibrillation, digoxin slows the heart beat.

Match the following.

1. ____ thrombocytopenia

2. ____ spironolactone

3. ____ captopril

4. ____ nesiritide

5. ____ digoxin

6. ____ pulse deficit

7. ____ photophobia

8. ____ furosemide

9. ____ pulmonary edema

10. ____ cough

a. A loop diuretic used in clients with heart failure who have impaired renal function

b. Occurs when left ventricular failure causes blood to accumulate in pulmonary veins and tissues

c. Drug of choice to treat clients who have chronic heart failure

d. The only commonly used digitalis glycoside

e. An adverse effect of prolonged use of inamrinone

f. A characteristic of moderate or severe heart failure

g. An aldosterone antagonist used in moderate to severe heart failure

h. Used in the management of acute heart failure to increase diuresis and secretion of sodium and decrease the secretion of neurohormones

i. Faster apical rate than radial rate

j. An adverse effect of digoxin

■ Clinical Challenge

A client, a 70-year-old female, is admitted to the coronary care unit complaining of nausea and vomiting. She has a heart rate of 46 beats per minute. Initial assessment reveals that she is currently taking digoxin, furosemide, and a potassium supplement. A diagnosis of digoxin toxicity is made according to serum digoxin concentrations. With this diagnosis, what will the nurse monitor throughout the client's stay in the unit? What is the therapeutic range of digoxin the nurse will be looking for?

After several days in the unit, the client's serum digoxin is within the therapeutic range. She is to be discharged on Lanoxin 0.125 mg PO daily. What will the nurse include in client instruction regarding the medication?

The client asks the nurse why her heart rate was so slow. How should the nurse respond?

■ Review Questions

1. Your client has been successfully digitalized. Serum levels of digoxin are within therapeutic range. The nurse will monitor which of the following to determine the maintenance dose of digoxin?

   a. hepatic function

   b. creatinine clearance

   c. potassium levels

   d. magnesium levels

2. A 72-year-old male is admitted to the cardiac care unit with severe heart failure. He is to receive a bolus dose of inamirone (Inacor). The nurse will observe for which of the following adverse effects?

   a. dysrhythmias

   b. headache

   c. disorientation

   d. seizures

3. A client is to be discharged on Lanoxin 0.125 mg daily. Which of the following statements by the client indicates successful client teaching by the nurse?

   a. "If I miss a dose, I should not take 2 tablets in 1 day."

   b. "I will have to take this drug 2 or 3 months."

   c. "This drug can cause a bitter taste in my mouth."

   d. "This drug may cause me to retain fluid."

4. The nurse is monitoring a client's serum digoxin levels and is aware that the therapeutic range is:

   a. 0.125 to 0.5 ng/mL

   b. 0.2 to 1.0 ng/mL

   c. 0.5 to 2.0 ng/mL

   d. 3.5 to 5.0 ng/mL

5. A nursing action related to the care of a client who is receiving digoxin includes:

   a. administering the drug subcutaneously

   b. relying on client blood pressure readings for dosage

   c. reporting an apical heart rate below 60 to the client's physician

   d. discontinuing the medication if the serum digoxin level is within therapeutic range

6. A 58-year-old male is admitted to the emergency room. A diagnosis of severe digoxin toxicity is made. Which of the following drugs may be given immediately?

   a. digoxin immune fab

   b. furosemide

   c. captopril

   d. dopamine

7. Your client is taking digoxin (Lanoxin) 0.125 mg daily for heart failure. She reports to you that since she has been on the drug, she can breathe better and her heart rate has been around 74 beats per minute. You also notice that, according to the scales, she has lost 3 pounds since her last visit. You suspect that:

   a. the drug dosage will be increased

   b. the drug dosage will stay the same

   c. the drug dosage will be decreased

   d. the drug will be discontinued

8. Which of the following should be emphasized when instructing a client who is to begin taking digoxin (Lanoxin)?

   a. Digoxin tablets may be crushed and taken with food.

   b. Digoxin should not be taken with an antacid.

   c. It doesn't matter what time of day digoxin is taken.

   d. If a daily dose is missed, it may be taken with the next dose.

9. Which of the following indicates a therapeutic effect of digoxin (Lanoxin) when given for an atrial dsyrhythmia?

   a. increase in weight

   b. elimination of pulse deficit

   c. gradual increase in heart rate

   d. decrease in edema

10. Your client is to receive nesiritide (Natrecor) for acute heart failure. It is important for the nurse to remember that:

    a. the drug must be administered through a separate IV line

    b. a bolus injection of Natrecor must be given over a 10-minute period

    c. the drug cannot be diluted with sodium chloride

    d. it is not necessary to prime the infusion tubing prior to administration

CHAPTER 52

Antidysrhythmic Drugs

■ Exercises

Fill in the blank.

1. Electrical impulses in the heart depend on the movement of _____ and _____ ions into a myocardial cell and movement of _____ ions out of the cell.

2. Activation of the SA node depends on a slow depolarizing current through _____ channels.

3. Rapid depolarizing current through _____ channels activate the atria and ventricles.

4. The ability of a cardiac muscle cell to respond to an electrical stimulus is called _____.

5. The period following contraction when the cell cannot respond to a new stimulus is called the _____ _____ period.

6. The period before the resting membrane potential is reached and a stimulus greater than normal is needed to produce a response is called _____ _____ period.

7. _____ is the ability of cardiac tissue to transmit electrical impulses.

8. Cardiac dysrhythmias result from _____ in electrical impulses.

9. _____ increases myocardial irritability and is considered a risk factor for atrial and ventricular dysrhythmias.

10. _____ _____ is the most common dysrhythmia.

11. _____ is the only FDA-approved antidysrhythmic drug for children.

12. _____ _____ are the most common sustained dysrhythmias in children.

13. _____ tachycardia is characterized by three or more premature ventricular contractions occurring in a row at a rate greater than 100 beats per minute.

14. Three nonpharmacologic methods for management of dysrhythmias include _____ _____ _____ _____, _____ _____, and _____.

15. Abnormal electrical impulses (ectopic foci) may be activated by _____, _____, and _____ or _____ _____.

Complete the chart.

Drug	Dysrhythmia use	Classification	Therapeutic level	Adverse effects
lidocaine				
quinidine				
verapamil				
amiodarone				
disopyramide				

Match the following.

1. ____ tocainide (Tonocard)

2. ____ flecainide (Tambocor)

3. ____ lidocaine (Xylocaine)

4. ____ moricizine (Ethmozine)

5. ____ ibutilide (Corvert)

6. ____ phenytoin (Dilantin)

7. ____ quinidine (Quinaglute)

8. ____ amiodarone (Cordarone)

9. ____ procainamide (Pronestyl)

10 ____ acebutolol (Sectral)

a. When used long term, may increase the effects of anticoagulants

b. Prototype of class IB antidysrhythmias; must be given by injection

c. Can cause new dysrhythmias or aggravate preexisting dysrhythmias

d. Anticonvulsant used to treat dysrhythmias

e. Indicated for recent onset of atrial fibrillation or atrial flutter

f. Adverse effects include a syndrome similar to lupus erythematosus

g. Prototype for class IA antidysrhythmias; use is declining

h. Used for chronic therapy to prevent ventricular dysrhythmias precipitated by exercise

i. Recommended for use only in life-threatening ventricular dysrhythmias

j. Oral analog of lidocaine

■ Clinical Challenge

A 79-year-old client is admitted to the emergency room with severe chest pain. He is diaphoretic and complaining of shortness of breath and nausea. The cardiac monitor reveals sinus tachycardia and frequent premature ventricular complexes. He is to receive an IV lidocaine bolus. How much lidocaine will the nurse prepare? How will the medication be administered? After the bolus dose, the nurse will maintain a continuous infusion of lidocaine at what rate? How will the nurse monitor the lidocaine levels?

What does the nurse need to know about mixing other drugs with lidocaine? What side effects will the nurse observe for?

■ Review Questions

1. A client has been diagnosed with paroxysmal supraventricular tachycardia. He is started on verapamil (Calan). The nurse will assess for which of the following?
   a. headache
   b. diarrhea
   c. constipation
   d. muscle and joint pain

2. Your client is to receive disopyramide (Norpace). The nurse should assess for which of the following conditions?
   a. hepatic disease
   b. peptic ulcer disease
   c. seizure disorder
   d. renal insufficiency

3. The expected outcome for a client who is taking an antidysrhythmic drug would be:
   a. increased cardiac output
   b. decreased cardiac output
   c. increased renal insufficiency
   d. decreased respiratory distress

4. Your client is being discharged from the hospital on an antidysrhythmic drug. It is important that the client/caregiver report which of the following?
   a. dizziness
   b. constipation
   c. increased appetite
   d. stiffness in joints

5. Before administering an antidysrhythmic drug, the nurse should:
   a. take the client's temperature
   b. assess the client's mental status
   c. check the apical and radial pulses
   d. place the client in semi-Fowler's position

6. Your client has been on disopyramide (Norpace) for 3 days. You will assess for which of the following adverse effects?
   a. increased blood pressure
   b. dry mouth
   c. edema
   d. severe diarrhea

7. The heart monitor indicates that your client is experiencing supraventricular tachycardia. You are to administer diltiazem (Cardizem) 20 mg IV push. During the administration of this drug you will observe for:
   a. decreased heart rate
   b. increased heart rate
   c. increased blood pressure
   d. increased body temperature

8. Verapamil (Calan) is contraindicated in a client who has:
   a. diabetes mellitus
   b. respiratory impairment
   c. digoxin toxicity
   d. edema

9. Which of the following instructions should be given to a client who is taking quinidine (Quinaglute)?
   a. Decrease salt intake.
   b. Take the medication with orange juice.
   c. Decrease the fiber in diet.
   d. Take the medication with meals.

10. A client is taking propranolol (Inderal) for a dysrhythmia. The client should be instructed to:
    a. report a weight gain of over 2 pounds
    b. increase caloric intake
    c. have her blood pressure checked every day
    d. observe for blood in her urine

■Cardiac Electrophysiology Diagram, Part I

Fill in the blanks in Figure 52-1 with the terms below to identify the components of the heart's conduction system.

AV junction
Purkinje fibers
Inferior branch of left
    bundle branch
SA node

Anterior branch of left
    bundle branch
Bundle of His
AV node

Main stem of left
    bundle branch
Internodal tracts
Right bundle branch
Intra-atrial tract

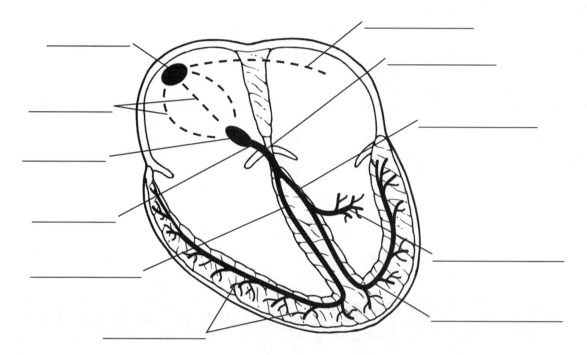

FIGURE 52-1.

▪Cardiac Electrophysiology Diagram, Part II

Use the Diagram Completion answers from Part I of this exercise to complete the following sentences.

1. Verapamil, a calcium channel blocker, is used to treat supraventricular tachycardia and atrial fibrillation and flutter because it slows conduction through the _____ and _____.

2. Atropine is the drug of choice for heart block because it improves conduction through the _____, and increases conduction through these parts of the heart: _____, _____, _____, _____, and _____.

3. Disopyramide (Norpace), given orally to adults to treat ventricular tachyarrhythmias, works by reducing automaticity in the _____ node, slowing conduction through the _____ node, and prolonging the refractory period.

▪Dysrhythmia Analysis

Select the appropriate term from the list below to pair each of the dysrhythmias with a drug that might be ordered for its treatment.

Digoxin (Lanoxin)
Lidocaine (Xylocaine)
Supraventricular tachycardia
Adenosine (Adenocard)

Atrial fibrillation
Sinus bradycardia
Atropine
Premature ventricular contractions

1. Dysrhythmia _____ Treatment _____

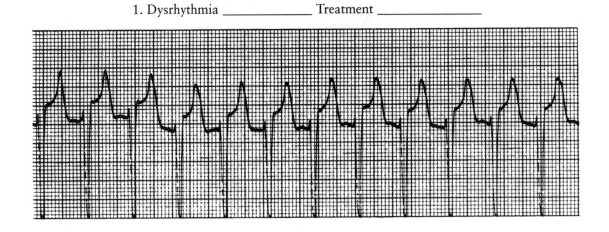

2. Dysrhythmia _____ Treatment _____

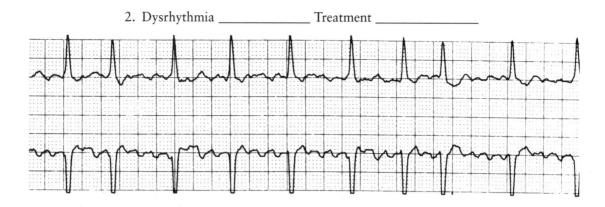

3. Dysrhythmia _____ Treatment _____

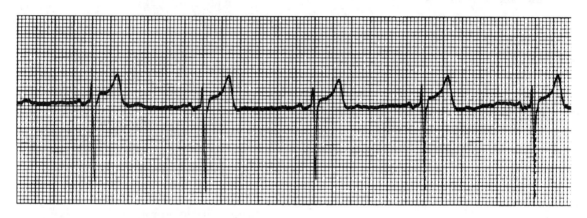

4. Dysrhythmia _____ Treatment _____

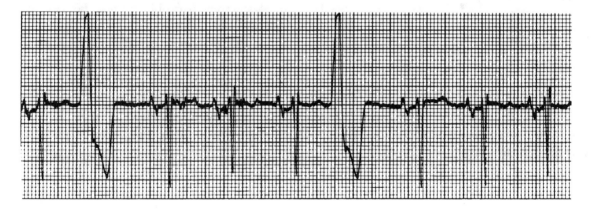

CHAPTER 53

Antianginal Drugs

■ Exercises

Answer the following.

1. What causes angina pectoris to develop?

2. Describe the development of coronary artery disease.

3. List the three main types of angina.

4. Describe anginal pain.

5. When coronary atherosclerosis develops slowly, why does collateral circulation develop?

6. List the drugs used for myocardial ischemia.

Match the following.

1. ____ Beta-adrenergic blocking agents

2. ____ nifedipine (Procardia)

3. ____ nadolol (Corgard)

4. ____ aspirin

5. ____ nitroglycerin

6. ____ cimetidine

7. ____ isosorbide mononitrate (Ismo)

8. ____ carbamazepine (Tegretol)

9. ____ propranolol (Inderal)

10. ____ isosorbide dinitrate (Isordil)

a. The prototype beta blocker

b. Organic nitrate prototype

c. Used in long-term management of angina to decrease frequency and severity of attacks

d. Has become part of the standard of care in coronary heart disease

e. Beta-adrenergic blocker that can be given once daily

f. Used only for prophylaxis of angina

g. The prototype of the dihydropyridine group of calcium channel-blocking agent

h. Decreases effects of calcium channel blockers

i. Effective oral dose obtained by increasing the dose until headache occurs

j. Increases beta-blocking effect of propranolol

Place a T (true) or F (false) in each blank.

1. ____ The most common causes of angina are low blood pressure and an increased amount of blood and oxygen to the heart.

2. ____ Long-acting medications for angina are not effective in relieving sudden anginal pain.

3. ____ Clients may increase or decrease dosages of medication for angina according to frequency and severity of attacks.

4. ____ Nitroglycerin tablets should be replaced every 6 months.

5. ____ Hypertension is an adverse effect of antianginal drugs.

6. ____ A health care provider should always wear gloves when applying nitroglycerin ointment.

7. ____ Nitroglycerin patches may be applied anywhere on the body.

8. ____ It takes between 3 and 5 hours for transmucosal tablets to dissolve.

9. ____ Bradycardia is an adverse effect of nitrates.

10. ____ Nifedipine (Procardia) may cause hypotension.

■ Clinical Challenge

The client is a 43-year-old male who is admitted to the hospital with increasing episodes of angina with minimal exertion. He is to begin isosorbide dinitrate sustained-release 40-mg tablets. What would be the nurse's instructions regarding administration of this drug?

The client shows no improvement in 12 hours. The physician orders nifedipine (Procardia) 10 mg PO every 6 hours. Why will the nurse monitor the client for hypotension?

The client begins to show improvement and is ready for discharge. What instructions will the nurse give to the client?

■ Review Questions

1. Your client is admitted to the hospital with a diagnosis of chest pain. He has an order for nitroglycerin 0.3 mg SL PRN for chest pain. Which of the following actions should you do when he complains of chest pain?
   a. Call the physician.
   b. Place 3 nitroglycerin tablets under his tongue.
   c. Have the client swallow a tablet every 5 minutes for 20 minutes.
   d. Administer a tablet under his tongue; may need to repeat in 5 minutes and again in 5 more minutes.

2. Which of the following would indicate a contraindication for the use of nitroglycerin?
   a. a client with hypertension
   b. a client with severe anemia
   c. a client with thyroid disease
   d. a client with diabetes mellitus

3. An expected outcome for a client who has just taken nitroglycerin should be:
   a. increased pulse and decreased blood pressure
   b. decreased pulse and decreased blood pressure
   c. increased pulse and increased blood pressure
   d. decreased pulse and increased blood pressure

4. The nurse explains to the client that nitroglycerin patches should be applied in the morning and removed in the evening. This dosage schedule reduces:
   a. nitrate tolerance
   b. adverse effects
   c. toxic effects
   d. nitrate dependence

5. The most common adverse effect of nitroglycerin is:
   a. diuresis
   b. pounding headache
   c. irritability
   d. dry mouth

6. Which of the following conditions would a nurse assess for before starting nifedipine (Procardia) therapy?
   a. severe hepatic disease
   b. Raynaud's syndrome
   c. diabetes mellitus
   d. myasthenia gravis

7. Your client complains of headaches and dizziness with nitrate therapy. Which of the following would be the most appropriate response to her?
   a. "Avoid strenuous activity and stand up slowly."
   b. "These effects are temporary and should subside with continuous use."
   c. "You will have these adverse effects as long as you use nitroglycerin."
   d. "You may reduce your dosage to help relieve the adverse effects."

8. Your client has started nitrate antianginal therapy. When discussing dizziness, you will instruct him to avoid:
   a. a high-fat diet
   b. alcohol
   c. dairy products
   d. over-the-counter cold remedies

9. In regard to the administration of oral nitrates, the nurse will instruct the client to:
   a. take on an empty stomach
   b. take with food
   c. place the tablet between the cheek and gum
   d. place the tablet under the tongue

10. You are applying a topical preparation of nitroglycerin. Your *initial* action will be to:
    a. place the ointment on a nonhairy part of the body
    b. wipe off the previous dose
    c. cover the area with a plastic wrap or tape
    d. put on a pair of gloves

CHAPTER 54

Drugs Used in Hypotension and Shock

■ Exercises

Match the following.

1. ____ septic shock

2. ____ hypovolemic shock

3. ____ anaphylactic shock

4. ____ neurogenic shock

5. ____ distributive shock

6. ____ cardiogenic shock

a. Can result from any organisms that enter the bloodstream

b. Results from hypersensitivity

c. Characterized by severe vasodilation, which results in severe hypotension and impairment of blood flow

d. Results from inadequate sympathetic nervous system stimulation

e. Involves a loss of intravascular fluid volume

f. Occurs when the myocardium has lost its ability to contract efficiently and maintain adequate cardiac output

Fill in the blank.

1. Drugs used in the management of shock are primarily _____ drugs.

2. _____ is a naturally occurring catecholamine that is useful in hypovolemic and cardiogenic shock.

3. _____ is the drug of choice for management of anaphylactic shock.

4. _____ is used only in shock associated with decreased heart rates and myocardial depression.

5. _____ is used mainly in hypotension occurring from spinal anesthesia.

6. _____ is used mainly in clients who do not respond to dopamine or dobutamine.

7. _____ and _____ are most often the cardiotonic drugs used in critically ill clients.

8. _____ is the drug of first choice in distributive shock.

9. _____ is less likely to cause tachycardia and dysrhythmias than are dopamine and isoproterenol.

10. _____ decreases the effectiveness of dopamine.

■ Clinical Challenge

Your client is in the cardiac care unit with a diagnosis of cardiogenic shock. He is getting dopamine (Intropin) intravenously. What will dopamine do for this client? Why is adequate fluid therapy necessary for this client?

■ Review Questions

1. You are starting an IV on a client who is to receive IV dopamine (Intropin). To decrease the risk of extravasation, you will:

   a. administer a concentrated solution of dopamine

   b. dilute the dopamine in 50 mL of IV fluids

   c. use a large vein for the venipuncture site

   d. mix the dopamine with other drugs to be administered

2. You have started an IV dopamine (Intropin) drip. The flow rate will be titrated according to:

   a. the client's response to the drug

   b. the manufacturer's directions

   c. the weight of the client

   d. the type of shock the client is experiencing

3. Your client has been receiving dopamine (Intropin) for the management of hypovolemia. The physician has discontinued the drug. You will stop the drug gradually in order to prevent:

   a. hypertension

   b. hypotension

   c. dysrhythmia

   d. tachycardia

4. An expected client outcome of drug therapy for hypotension associated with shock is:

   a. systolic blood pressure of 180 and heart rate of 40

   b. systolic blood pressure of 80 and heart rate of 120

   c. systolic blood pressure of 98 and heart rate of 70

   d. systolic blood pressure of 130 and heart rate of 50

5. Extravasation of dopamine (Intropin) has occurred with your client. Which of the following drugs will you administer?

   a. diltiazem (Cardizem)

   b. phentolamine (Regitine)

   c. cinoxacin (Cinobac)

   d. betamethasone (Celestone)

6. Which of the following is the most important nursing measure when caring for a client who is being managed for shock?

   a. Monitor blood pressure frequently.

   b. Take apical pulse prior to medication administration.

   c. Weigh daily.

   d. Decrease fluid intake.

7. You are caring for a critically ill client who is receiving epinephrine. You are aware that the recommended infusion rate will be between:

   a. 0.002 to 0.01 mcg/kg/min

   b. 0.01 to 0.15 mcg/kg/min

   c. 0.02 to 0.2 mcg/kg/min

   d. 0.1 to 1.0 mcg/kg/min

8. Dopamine (Intropin) is being given to your client who is experiencing cardiogenic shock. Which of the following is necessary for a maximum therapeutic effect of the drug?

   a. administration of a cardiac glycoside

   b. a heart rate above 50

   c. an infusion rate of 100 μg/kg/min

   d. adequate fluid therapy

9. Which of the following decreases the effectiveness of dopamine (Intropin)?

   a. acidosis

   b. alkalosis

   c. benign prostatic hypertrophy

   d. hypokalemia

10. Your client is receiving isoproterenol (Isuprel) in the management of shock. You will be aware of the following adverse effect?

    a. bradycardia

    b. tachycardia

    c. hypotension

    d. acidosis

CHAPTER 55

Antihypertensive Drugs

■ Exercises

Place a T (true) or F (false) in each blank.

1. ____ Hypertension is defined as a systolic pressure above 160 mm Hg or a diastolic pressure above 100 mm Hg on more than one blood pressure measurement.

2. ____ It is best to lower blood pressure gradually.

3. ____ Captopril (Capoten) is recommended as a first-line agent for treating hypertension in diabetic clients.

4. ____ Angiotensin II receptor blockers are more likely to cause hyperkalemia than are angiotensin-converting enzyme (ACE) inhibitors.

5. ____ Vasodilator antihypertensive drugs directly relax smooth muscle in blood vessels to decrease peripheral vascular resistance.

6. ____ Children have a greater incidence of secondary hypertension than do adults.

7. ____ Captopril (Capoten) is a first-line agent for children with hypertension.

8. ____ A diuretic is the drug of first choice in older adults who are hypertensive.

9. ____ ACE inhibitors are used to help diabetic clients with renal impairment.

10. ____ Nonprescription medication may decrease the effectiveness of antihypertensive drugs.

Match the following

1. ____ captopril (Capoten)

2. ____ verapamil (Calan)

3. ____ nifedipine (Procardia)

4. ____ losartan (Cozaar)

5. ____ clonidine (Catapres)

6. ____ fenoldopam (Corlopam)

7. ____ hydrochlorothiazide

8. ____ prazosin (Minipress)

9. ____ sodium nitroprusside (Nipride)

10. ____ propranolol (Inderal)

a. Decreases renin release from the kidneys to decrease blood pressure

b. May cause orthostatic hypotension with palpitations

c. A short-acting calcium channel blocker used to treat hypertensive emergencies or urgencies

d. The first angiotensin II receptor blocker that may be used in combination with hydrochlorothiazide

e. A thiazide diuretic commonly used to treat hypertension

f. A vasodilator that acts on arterioles and venules to decrease blood pressure

g. Initial dose may be taken at bedtime to prevent acute hypotension

h. A fast-acting drug indicated for short-term use in hypertensive emergencies

i. Considered as an alpha$_2$ receptor agonist

j. A calcium channel blocker that dilates peripheral arteries and decreases peripheral vascular resistance by relaxing vascular smooth muscle to decrease blood pressure

■ Discussion

Describe the three mechanisms that regulate blood pressure.

Answer the following.

1. List nonpharmacologic measures to control hypertension.

2. List conditions that may cause a person to be at risk for hypertension.

■ Clinical Challenge

Your client, age 69, is admitted to the intensive care unit in hypertensive crisis. Her blood pressure at time of admission is 225/160 mm Hg. She is to receive nitroprusside (Nipride) IV. At what rate will you infuse the medication? What is the expected outcome of the Nipride therapy?

After a day of therapy, your client develops slurred speech and muscle twitching, and has a seizure. What should you do regarding Nipride therapy?

■ Review Questions

1. A client has been placed on captopril (Capoten) PO 25 mg BID. The nurse should instruct the client to:
   a. avoid citric juices with administration of the drug
   b. take the medication with a full glass of water
   c. take the medication on an empty stomach
   d. take the medication with food

2. Clonidine (Catapres) skin patches are applied to a hairless area on the upper arm or torso how often?
   a. every day
   b. every other day
   c. every 3 days
   d. every 7 days

3. The physician has prescribed prazosin (Minipress) 1 mg PO daily. When teaching the client about this drug, the nurse will stress:
   a. taking the first dose at bedtime to prevent dizziness
   b. limiting fluid intake to 1000 mL per day to decrease urinary output
   c. taking the drug early in the day to prevent sleepiness
   d. taking the drug on an empty stomach to promote absorption

4. The nurse is planning follow-up care for a client who has been taking hydrochlorothiazide (HydroDiuril) for hypertension. An additional antihypertensive agent has been added to her treatment regimen. The nurse is aware that:
   a. most clients on multidrug therapy follow the treatment plan
   b. most clients understand the importance of taking their medication as prescribed
   c. clients who are actively involved in their therapy are usually more compliant
   d. it is unusual for more than one medication to be prescribed for hypertension

5. In determining whether a client can be started on metoprolol (Lopressor), the nurse may question the client concerning:

 a. renal disease

 b. hepatic disease

 c. diabetes mellitus

 d. peptic ulcer disease

6. Your client has a prescription for ramipril (Altace). She asks you how long it will take to lower her blood pressure. The most appropriate response to her would be:

 a. "That's a question you should really ask your doctor."

 b. "It will probably take 3 to 4 weeks before you feel better."

 c. "This drug usually produces effects within 1 hour after you take a dose."

 d. "It will take 6 months before you feel any effects of the drug."

7. Your client is diabetic and has been diagnosed with hypertension. An ACE inhibitor has been prescribed for her. Which of the following may develop as a result of the drug therapy?

 a. hypocalcemia

 b. hypercalcemia

 c. hypokalemia

 d. hyperkalemia

8. A 62-year-old female is taking losartan (Cozaar) for hypertension. It has been determined that the drug therapy is not controlling her blood pressure. Which of the following drugs may be added to her treatment plan?

 a. hydrochlorothiazide

 b. omeprazole

 c. fenoldopam

 d. nitroprusside

9. Chronic use of clonidine may result in:

 a. vertigo

 b. irritability

 c. nausea

 d. sodium and fluid retention

10. Your client is a 42-year-old African American male who has been diagnosed with hypertension. You suspect the doctor will prescribe:

 a. a calcium channel blocker

 b. a diuretic

 c. a beta blocker

 d. an ACE inhibitor

CHAPTER 56

Diuretics

■ Exercises

Fill in the blank.

1. The main function of the kidneys is to regulate the _____, _____, and _____ of body fluids.

2. The functional unit of the kidney is the _____.

3. Each nephron is composed of a _____ and a _____.

4. Most reabsorption occurs in the _____ _____.

5. Secretion of _____ _____ is necessary in maintaining acid-base balance in body fluids.

6. _____ is the excessive accumulation of fluid in body tissues.

7. The tubules are described as _____ because of their many twists and turns.

8. Movement of substances from the glomerular filtrate to blood in the peritubular capillaries is called _____.

9. _____ is reabsorbed in the descending limb of the Henle's loop.

10. _____ promotes sodium-potassium exchange in the distal tubule and collecting ducts.

Match the following.

1. ____ spironolactone (Aldactone)

2. ____ hyperkalemia

3. ____ torsemide (Demadex)

4. ____ hydrochlorothiazide (HydroDIURIL)

5. ____ mannitol (Osmitrol)

6. ____ ototoxicity

7. ____ hypokalemia

8. ____ chlorothiazide (Diuril)

9. ____ pulmonary edema

10. ____ furosemide (Lasix)

a. An osmotic agent

b. Prototype for loop diuretics

c. May occur with potassium-losing diuretics

d. Adverse effect likely to occur with furosemide

e. Only thiazide diuretic that can be given IV

f. Adverse effect that occurs with osmotic diuretics

g. May be taken without regard to meals

h. Blocks the sodium-retaining effects of aldosterone

i. Major adverse effect of potassium-sparing diuretics

j. Most commonly used thiazide diuretic

Place a T (true) or F (false) in each blank.

1. ____ Diuretics decrease renal excretion of water, sodium, and other electrolytes.

2. ____ Each kidney contains approximately 100 nephrons.

3. ____ Sodium is reabsorbed in the ascending limb of Henle's loop.

4. ____ Edema interferes with blood flow to tissues.

5. ____ Initially, diuretics increase blood volume and cardiac output.

6. ____ Furosemide (Lasix) is contraindicated in a client who is allergic to sulfonamide drugs.

7. ____ Dietary sodium is restricted in loop diuretic therapy.

8. ____ Loop diuretics are the drugs of choice when rapid diuresis is required.

9. ____ Furosemide (Lasix) is the loop diuretic most often used in children.

10. ____ Bumetanide (Bumex) produces less ototoxicity than does furosemide.

■ Clinical Challenge

Your client is admitted to the intensive care unit with symptoms of pulmonary edema and impaired renal function. IV furosemide (Lasix) is started. Because of the client's kidney disease, you will monitor which values? Which adverse effect will you also assess for?

Your client continues to improve and is discharged after several days. PO furosemide has been ordered. What will you include in your teaching plan when he is discharged?

■ Review Questions

1. A client is being treated for mild hypertension with chlorothiazide (Diuril) 500 mg PO daily. The nurse will teach her about which of the following adverse effects?
   a. muscle cramps
   b. drowsiness
   c. nausea and vomiting
   d. dry mouth

2. A 48-year-old female is diabetic and has been on oral hypoglycemics for several years. She has recently been diagnosed with hypertension and started on a thiazide diuretic. The nurse is aware that the diuretic may cause which of the following?
   a. hypoglycemia
   b. hyperglycemia
   c. hypokalemia
   d. hyperkalemia

3. The most appropriate nursing intervention for a client who is hospitalized and has just begun diuretic therapy would be to:
   a. record blood pressure readings two to four times daily
   b. weigh the client every other day
   c. record fluid intake and output every 36 hours
   d. enforce strict bedrest

4. To avoid increased risks of adverse effects, the nurse will administer an IV injection of furosemide over:
   a. 1 to 2 minutes
   b. 2 to 3 minutes
   c. 2 to 5 minutes
   d. 5 minutes

5. For clients at home, oral diuretics should be taken:
   a. early in the morning
   b. at noon
   c. during the afternoon hours
   d. at bedtime

6. Your client is taking an antihypertensive agent and a diuretic. You will teach him to:
   a. take both drugs on an empty stomach
   b. suck on hard candy
   c. change positions slowly
   d. increase daily exercise

7. A client is taking a potassium-sparing diuretic. Which of the following instructions should the nurse give to her?
   a. "Decrease salt in your diet."
   b. "Limit your intake of foods high in potassium."
   c. "Drink two glasses of orange juice and eat a banana every day."
   d. "Decrease fat in your diet."

8. A 16-year-old boy is admitted to the intensive care unit with increased intracranial pressure from a head injury. Which of the following diuretics will be administered to him?
   a. furosemide (Lasix)
   b. chlorothiazide (Diuril)
   c. spironolactone (Aldactone)
   d. mannitol (Osmitrol)

9. Your client is taking hydrochlorothiazide (HydroDIURIL) for ankle edema. On a follow-up visit to the clinic, she states that she has taken her medication as prescribed but continues to have swelling. You should assess for:

   a. alcohol intake

   b. sodium intake in her diet

   c. activity level

   d. possible drug–drug interactions

10. Your client has been on hydrochlorothiazide (HydroDIURIL) therapy for 3 weeks. Which of the following serum potassium levels indicate she is experiencing hypokalemia?

    a. 2.8 mEq/L

    b. 3.9 mEq/L

    c. 4.1 mEq/L

    d. 5 mEq/L

■ Nephron Diagram

Fill in the blanks in Figure 56-1 with the terms below.

Descending limb of Henle's loop
Glomerulus
Ascending limb of Henle's loop
Henle's loop
Efferent arteriole
Bowman's capsule
Afferent arteriole
Distal tubule
Collecting tubule
Proximal tubule

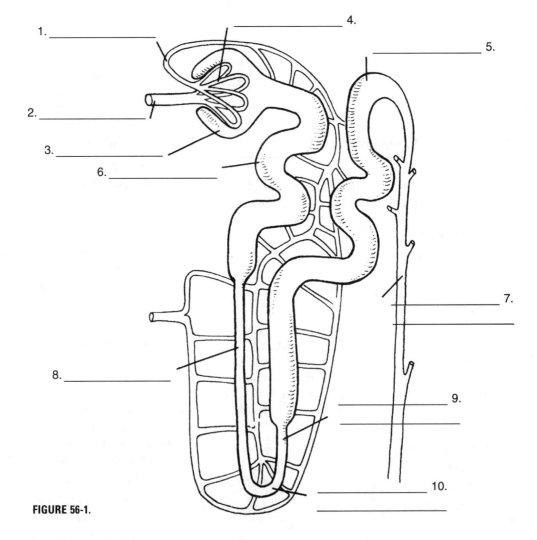

FIGURE 56-1.

CHAPTER 57

Drugs That Affect Blood Coagulation

■ Exercises

Fill in the blank.

1. _____ involves the formation or presence of a blood clot in a blood vessel.

2. An _____ is part of a thrombus that breaks off and travels to another part of the body.

3. Pathologic thrombosis is often the result of _____.

4. A thrombus may precipitate _____ _____.

5. _____ is the prevention of blood loss from an injured blood vessel.

Place a T (true) or F (false) in each blank.

1. ____ Blood clotting is a normal body defense mechanism.

2. ____ Anticoagulants are more effective in preventing arterial thrombosis than venous thrombosis.

3. ____ Anticoagulant drugs dissolve formed clots.

4. ____ Heparin does not cross the placental barrier.

5. ____ Heparin is the most commonly used oral anticoagulant.

6. ____ Warfarin is contraindicated during pregnancy.

7. ____ Lepirudin is used as a heparin substitute.

8. ____ Heparin and warfarin are given during thrombolytic therapy.

9. ____ Protamine sulfate is an antidote for heparin.

10. ____ Ginkgo can decrease the effects of warfarin.

Indicate whether the drug increases or decreases the effect of warfarin by placing a check in the appropriate column.

Drug	Increases	Decreases
acetaminophen		
griseofulvin		
carbamazepine		
tetracycline		
furosemide		
fluconazole		
rifampin		
estrogen		
aspirin		
quinidine		

■ Clinical Challenge

Your client is a 32-year-old nursing student who develops deep vein thrombosis (DVT) in her left leg. She is hospitalized, and an initial assessment reveals that she has been on birth control pills for 3 months. She is to receive IV heparin, 30 units/kg of body weight on admission and 20,000 units every 24 hours by IV infusion. Bedrest is ordered. Why is heparin the drug of choice for your client? Which laboratory tests will be ordered for her, and how often will it be done? Why will you monitor her response to the medication?

■ Review Questions

1. Your client is receiving intermittent IV doses of heparin. A nursing action related to heparin administration would be to:

   a. massage back and legs

   b. observe for signs and symptoms of hemorrhage

   c. ambulate client three times a day

   d. protect IV bag and tubing from the light

2. As a nurse, you would know to have which of the following drugs available when a client is on heparin therapy?

   a. vitamin K

   b. aminocaproic acid (Amicar)

   c. protamine sulfate

   d. tranexamic acid

3. Heparin is contraindicated in a client with:

   a. deep vein thrombosis

   b. cirrhosis

   c. peptic ulcer disease

   d. acute myocardial infarction

4. A client has started warfarin (Coumadin) therapy for deep vein thrombosis. She asks the nurse how long it will be before the drug starts breaking up the clots. The nurse's response should be:

   a. "I'm not sure, but I'll ask your doctor."

   b. "It will take about 3 to 5 days for the anticoagulant effects to occur."

   c. "We should be able to see positive results in 24 hours."

   d. "Anticoagulant effects will start immediately."

5. Your client is on continuous IV heparin therapy. What time should blood be drawn for the partial thromboplastin time?

   a. at any time

   b. 6 AM

   c. 12 noon

   d. 9 PM

6. Your client has intermittent claudication from peripheral vascular disease in both legs. She is taking cilostazol. Which of the following would be a desired outcome of drug therapy for her?

   a. decreased shortness of breath

   b. walking a quarter mile without leg pain

   c. decreased blood pressure

   d. participation in a 2-mile Heart Walk

7. A client is receiving warfarin (Coumadin). She should be scheduled for which of the following laboratory tests to monitor drug effectiveness?

   a. prothrombin time (PT) only

   b. international normalized ratio and PT

   c. activated partial thromboplastin time and PT

   d. international normalized ratio (INR) only

8. Your client is to receive heparin 5000 units SC. When administering this medication, you should:

   a. pull the skin tight with thumb and forefinger before injecting the medication

   b. aspirate the syringe for possible blood return

   c. massage the area for 1 minute once the medication is administered and the needle removed

   d. avoid aspirating the syringe and massaging the injection site

9. A client in the cardiac care unit is receiving an IV of streptokinase infusion for a suspected acute myocardial infarction. During the administration of this drug, the nurse will monitor the client for:

   a. headache

   b. skin rash

   c. dry mouth

   d. increased blood pressure

10. Your client is taking warfarin (Coumadin) for continued therapy for myocardial infarction. You observe that she has hematuria and gingival bleeding. You will plan to administer:

    a. vitamin K

    b. protamine sulfate

    c. aspirin

    d. alteplase

CHAPTER 58

Drugs for Dyslipidemia

■ Exercises

Fill in the blank.

1. Blood lipids include _____, _____, and
   _____.

2. Blood lipids are transported in plasma by
   _____.

3. _____ cholesterol is involved in the
   formation of atherosclerotic plaques.

4. Extremely high _____ levels are
   associated with acute pancreatitis.

5. The drug _____ can reduce low-density
   lipoprotein (LDL) cholesterol within 2 weeks.

6. _____ are useful for clients who have low
   high-density lipoprotein (HDL) cholesterol
   levels.

7. A _____ agent is recommended for single-drug
   therapy to lower cholesterol.

8. _____ is the preferred dyslipidemic for
   clients with diabetes mellitus.

9. _____ and _____ may cause
   hepatotoxicity.

10. _____ is a food source that is known to
    lower cholesterol.

Complete the chart.

Blood lipid	Desired level	Borderline level	High level
Triglycerides			
Total serum cholesterol			
LDL Cholesterol			
HDL Cholesterol			

Place a T (true) or F (false) in each blank.

1. ____ Drugs for dyslipidemia should be taken in the morning because more cholesterol is produced in the morning hours.

2. ____ Statin-type dyslipidemics may increase sensitivity to sunlight.

3. ____ Cholesterol is necessary for normal body functioning.

4. ____ HDL transports cholesterol away from arteries and back to the liver, where it is broken down.

5. ____ Type III dyslipidemia is characterized by lipid deposits in the feet, knees, and elbows.

6. ____ LDL cholesterol has protective effects against coronary heart disease.

7. ____ Fibrate agents may cause gallstones.

8. ____ Estrogen replacement therapy increases HDL cholesterol.

9. ____ Dyslipidemic drugs may be given to children younger than 10 years of age.

10. ____ Statins are contraindicated in clients with active liver disease.

■ Clinical Challenge

Your client is 42 years old and is in the clinic for his annual physical. It is determined that his total serum cholesterol is 330 mg/dL. He becomes very upset and reveals that his father died when he was 48 years old from a "heart attack." The doctor decides to place him on niacin and asks you to discuss lifestyle changes with him. Discuss your teaching plans. What teaching will be needed regarding his medication?

■ Review Questions

1. Which of the following clients receiving gemfibrozil (Lopid) needs special instruction?
   a. a 52-year-old male bus driver
   b. a 25-year-old housewife
   c. a 73-year-old retired female teacher
   d. a 42-year-old sales associate

2. A client who has hyperlipidemia and is taking lovastatin (Mevacor) should be instructed to take the medication:
   a. with the evening meal
   b. at 12 noon with lunch
   c. 2 hours after breakfast
   d. at 9 PM before bedtime

3. Your client has high cholesterol and triglycerides. Her health care provider has prescribed niacin (nicotinic acid). During a follow-up visit, she complains of skin flushing. An appropriate response to her would be:
   a. "This is an adverse effect that will continue as long as you take the medication."
   b. "Don't worry about it. It's really not that noticeable."
   c. "Take 325 mg of ASA 30 minutes prior to the niacin dose. This should decrease the flushing."
   d. "You need to stop the medication immediately. I will notify your physician."

4. Which of the following may be responsible for noncompliance with statin therapy in older adults?
   a. severe adverse effects
   b. cost of the medication
   c. bitter taste of the medication
   d. frequency of dosage

5. A client who is taking cholestyramine (Questran) will most likely experience which of the following adverse effects?
   a. headache
   b. rash
   c. diarrhea
   d. constipation

6. Which of the following drugs may decrease the effects of lovastatin (Mevacor)?

    a. antacids

    b. alcohol

    c. erythromycin

    d. niacin

7. A client is taking atorvastatin (Lipitor). Which of the following should **not** be ingested with the drug?

    a. sweet potatoes

    b. grapefruit juice

    c. peanuts

    d. canned tuna

8. Your client has been diagnosed with type IV dyslipidemia. Which of the following laboratory tests should be performed prior to and during therapy?

    a. creatinine clearance and specific gravity

    b. blood glucose level

    c. serum aspartate and alanine aminotransferase

    d. complete blood count

9. Fenofibrate (Tricor) is contraindicated in which of the following conditions?

    a. hepatotoxicity

    b. severe renal impairment

    c. diabetes mellitus

    d. peptic ulcer disease

10. Which of the following dyslipidemic agents would be prescribed for a diabetic client?

    a niacin (Nicotinic acid)

    b. gemfibrozil (Lopid)

    c. glycerin (Glycerol)

    d. triamterene (Dyrenium)

CHAPTER 59

Physiology of the Digestive System

■ Exercises

Match the following.

1. ____ esophagus
2. ____ gallbladder
3. ____ duodenum
4. ____ liver
5. ____ alimentary canal
6. ____ saliva
7. ____ stomach
8. ____ pancreas
9. ____ pepsin
10. ____ peristalsis

a. Propels food through gastrointestinal tract and mixes food with the digestive juices
b. A tube extending from the mouth to the anus
c. Secretes insulin and glucagon
d. Small pouch on underside of the liver that stores and concentrates bile
e. Stores fat-soluble vitamins
f. A 10-inch tube that conveys food from the pharynx to the stomach
g. Lubricates the food bolus and starts starch digestion
h. Major digestive enzyme in gastric juice
i. First 10 to 12 inches of the small intestine
j. Serves as a reservoir for food

Place a T (true) or F (false) in each blank.

1. ____ Drugs used in digestive disorders act only systemically.

2. ____ Stimulation of the parasympathetic nervous system decreases gastrointestinal motility and secretions.

3. ____ Blood flow increases during digestion.

4. ____ Most drugs are absorbed from the stomach.

5. ____ The stomach normally holds approximately 2000 mL.

6. ____ Fatty foods cause the stomach to empty quickly.

7. ____ Enterogastrone is a hormone produced when fats are present in the duodenum.

8. ____ The large intestine consists of the cecum, colon, rectum, and anus.

9. ____ The gallbladder releases bile when fats are present in the duodenum.

10. ____ The liver receives approximately 500 mL of blood per minute.

■ Review Questions

1. The stomach normally empties in about:
   a. 1 hour
   b. 2 hours
   c. 4 hours
   d. 6 hours

2. Excess glucose that cannot be converted to glycogen is converted to:
   a. amino acids
   b. proteins
   c. carbohydrates
   d. fat

3. When the liver is damaged, which of the following may accumulate in body fluids?
   a. hormones
   b. bile
   c. glucose
   d. fat

4. The formation of which of the following removes ammonia from body fluids?
   a. glycogen
   b. urea
   c. bile
   d. galactose

5. Which body organ produces about 20% of total body heat?
   a. stomach
   b. pancreas
   c. gallbladder
   d. liver

6. The major digestive enzyme in gastric juice is:
   a. trypsin
   b. pepsin
   c. amylase
   d. lipase

7. Which of the following stimulates secretion of pancreatic juices?
   a. gastrin
   b. chymotrypsin
   c. amino acids
   d. cholecystokinin

8. When fats are present in the stomach, the duodenal mucosa produces:
   a. pepsin
   b. enterogastrone
   c. insulin
   d. phospholipids

9. The substance that initiates the digestion of starch is:
   a. saliva
   b. mucus
   c. insulin
   d. bile

10. Most digestion and absorption occur in the:
    a. liver
    b. stomach
    c. small intestine
    d. large intestine

■Digestive System Diagram

Match the organ with its function by filling in the blanks in Figure 59-1 with the letters below.

A. Absorption of most oral medications takes place here.
B. Water is absorbed here.
C. Secretes enzymes necessary for digestion.
D. Most drugs are metabolized here.
E. Releases bile when fats are present in the intestine.
F. Starch digestion starts here.
G. Protein breakdown occurs here.

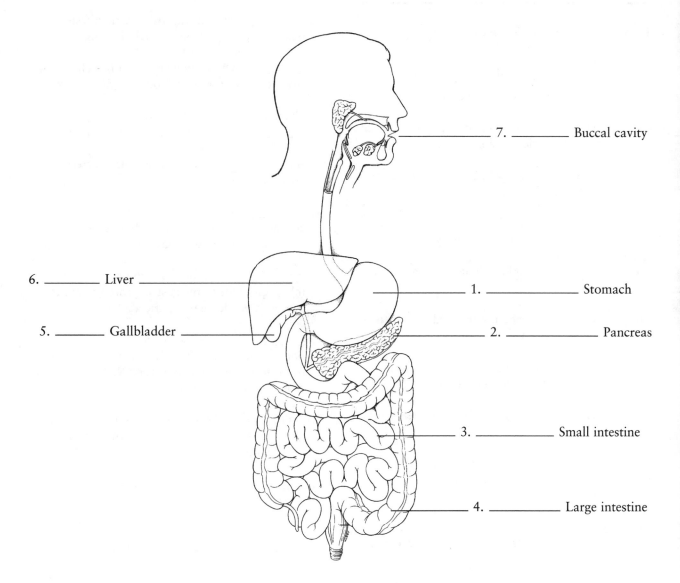

7. _____ Buccal cavity

6. _____ Liver

5. _____ Gallbladder

1. _____ Stomach

2. _____ Pancreas

3. _____ Small intestine

4. _____ Large intestine

FIGURE 59-1.

CHAPTER 60

Drugs Used in Peptic Ulcer and Acid Reflux Disorders

■ Exercises

Place a T (true) or F (false) in each blank.

1. _____ Gastric and duodenal ulcers are less common than esophageal ulcers.

2. _____ Pepsinogen is converted to pepsin when the pH of gastric juices is 3 or less.

3. _____ Smokers are more likely to develop duodenal ulcers.

4. _____ Gastroesophageal reflux disease (GERD) is common in people after 40 years of age.

5. _____ Antacids act primarily in the small intestine.

6. _____ Calcium compounds are used to treat peptic ulcer disease.

7. _____ Magnesium-based antacids are contraindicated in clients with renal failure.

8. _____ Cimetidine (Tagamet) is administered by the oral route only.

9. _____ Proton pump inhibitors are the drugs of first choice in most gastric and duodenal ulcers.

10. _____ Most cases of peptic ulcer disease are caused by a *Helicobactor pylori* infection.

Fill in the blank.

1. _____ ulcers most often are manifested by painless upper gastrointestinal bleeding.

2. _____ is a hormone released by cells in the stomach in response to food ingestion.

3. Commonly used antacids are _____, _____, and calcium compounds.

4. A _____ preparation exerts antibacterial effects against *H. pylori*.

5. _____ is more likely to cause mental confusion and gynecomastia than are other histamine-2 receptor antagonists.

6. _____, the first proton pump inhibitor, binds to the gastric proton pump to prevent the release of gastric acid.

7. _____ is used concurrently with nonsteroidal anti-inflammatory drugs (NSAIDs) to protect gastric mucosa from NSAID-induced erosion and ulceration.

8. A drug used in healing duodenal ulcers and in maintenance therapy to prevent the recurrence of ulcers is _____.

9. _____ increases blood level of diazepam.

10. _____ and _____ are contraindicated in clients with impaired renal function.

Match the following.

1. ____ pepsin

2. ____ gastric ulcers

3. ____ GERD

4. ____ proton pump inhibitors

5. ____ pyrosis

6. ____ gastritis

7. ____ gastropathy

8. ____ antacid

9. ____ *H. pylori*

10. ____ duodenal ulcers

a. Associated with stress, NSAID ingestion, and *H. pylori* infection; manifested by painless bleeding

b. Gram-negative bacterium found in the gastric mucosa

c. Strongest gastric acid suppressants

d. Proteolytic enzyme that helps digest protein foods

e. Acute gastritis resulting from irritation of the gastric mucosa

f. Caused by *H. pylori* infection and NSAID ingestion; associated with abdominal pain

g. An acute or chronic inflammatory reaction of gastric mucosa

h. Regurgitation of gastric content into the esophagus

i. Heartburn from gastroesophageal reflux disease (GERD)

j. An alkaline substance that neutralizes acids

■ Clinical Challenge

Your client is an 81-year-old male who was admitted to the hospital through the emergency department. He has been vomiting blood for the last 8 hours. Assessment data reveal that he has been taking prednisone, methotrexate, and Remicade for rheumatoid arthritis for the last 2 years. It is determined that he has a gastric ulcer. He is started on IV Protonix. After a weeklong stay in the hospital, the client is discharged and is to take Protonix PO. Why was Protonix ordered for this client? Identify adverse effects of Protonix. How

long do you suspect the client will have to take the medication? What instructions should be given to the client in regard to taking Protonix by mouth?

■ Review Questions

1. When teaching a client about taking antacids, the nurse will include which of the following information?

    a. Antacid tablets are not equal to the liquid form.

    b. Take antacids with food.

    c. Antacids absorb pepsin in the stomach.

    d. Do not take antacids with other medications.

2. Your client is taking sucralfate (Carafate). A potential nursing diagnosis for her would be:

    a. risk for constipation

    b. impaired urinary elimination

    c. activity intolerance

    d. deficient fluid volume

3. A 42-year-old male is being treated for a peptic ulcer with ranitidine (Zantac) 150 mg PO at bedtime. Even though few adverse effects have been associated with ranitidine, the nurse will inform the client of which of the following common adverse effects?

    a. headache

    b. irritability

    c. dry mouth

    d. fever

4. Your client is receiving drugs to prevent hyperacidity. An appropriate outcome for him would be:

    a. two formed stools per day

    b. loss of 2 pounds per week

    c. stools negative for occult blood

    d. increased appetite

5. Which of the following instructions would be given to a client in regard to administration of sucralfate (Carafate)?

   a. Take with meals.

   b. Take at least 1 hour before meals.

   c. Take after each meal.

   d. Take with a full glass of milk.

6. When evaluating a client on ranitidine therapy, which of the following laboratory tests should be performed?

   a. red blood cell count

   b. potassium level

   c. hepatic enzymes

   d. serum creatinine level

7. Your client is taking aluminum hydroxide. You expect the client to complain of:

   a. diarrhea

   b. constipation

   c. nausea

   d. headache

8. Your client is taking omeprazole (Prilosec). Which of the following is she being treated for?

   a. constipation

   b. GERD

   c. diarrhea

   d. asthma

9. A client has GERD and takes ranitidine (Zantac). She continues to have gastric discomfort and asks whether she can take an antacid. Your response should be:

   a. "Sure, you may take an antacid with Pepcid."

   b. "No, the two drugs will be working against each other."

   c. "Yes, but be sure to wait at least 1 hour to take the antacid after you take the Pepcid."

   d. "I wouldn't advise it. You may experience severe constipation."

10. Which of the following drugs would be indicated for a client who is taking NSAIDs for arthritis and is at high risk for gastrointestinal ulceration and bleeding?

    a. misoprostol (Cytotec)

    b. sucralfate (Carafate)

    c. lansoprazole (Prevacid)

    d. cimetidine (Tagamet)

CHAPTER 61

Laxatives and Cathartics

■ Exercises

Match the following agents to their characteristics and uses.

1. _____ act as a detergent to help mix fat and water in stools

2. _____ increase osmotic pressure in the intestinal lumen and cause water to be retained

3. _____ strongest and most abused laxative product

4. _____ most physiologic laxative

5. _____ used with caution in clients with congestive heart failure

6. _____ when water is added, these substances swell and become gel-like

7. _____ irritate the gastrointestinal (GI) mucosa and pull water into the bowel lumen

8. _____ used when rapid bowel evacuation is needed

9. _____ therapeutic effect is to prevent straining while expelling stool

10. _____ take 2 to 3 days to produce effects

11. _____ may produce serum electrolyte and acid-base imbalances with prolonged use

12. _____ lubricate fecal mass and slow colonic absorption of water

13. _____ stools have a semifluid consistency

14. _____ include castor oil

15. _____ effects may occur within ½ to 6 hours

a. Bulk-forming laxatives
b. Surfactant laxatives
c. Saline cathartics
d. Stimulant cathartics
e. Lubricant laxatives

Complete the chart by placing a check mark in a drug category for each drug.

Drug	Bulk-forming laxative	Surfactant laxative	Saline cathartic	Stimulant cathartic	Lubricant laxative
Mineral oil					
Dulcolax					
GoLYTELY					
Citrucel					
Mitrolan					
Castor oil					
Metamucil					
Milk of magnesia					
Colace					
Dialose					

■ Clinical Challenge

Your client is a 65-year-old female who is in the clinic for constipation. What would you tell her regarding risk factors for constipation? Other than the use of medication, what would you tell your client regarding prevention and treatment of constipation? Which drug do you suspect will be indicated for this client?

■ Review Questions

1. Your client has recently had a myocardial infarction. He is complaining of constipation. Which of the following drugs will be prescribed for him?
   a. methylcellulose (Citrucel)
   b. bisacodyl (Dulcolax)
   c. docusate sodium (Colace)
   d. castor oil (Neoloid)

2. You are caring for a 79-year-old male who has been in an extended care facility for 2 years. He has not had a bowel movement in 5 days. Before administering a laxative, you will check the client for:
   a. anxiety
   b. fecal impaction
   c. fever
   d. urinary incontinence

3. A client is to receive bisacodyl (Dulcolax) orally. The nurse will administer this drug with:
   a. food
   b. water
   c. milk
   d. antacid

4. You are instructing a client on the use of psyllium hydrophilic mucilloid. She asks you how long it will take to work. You will tell her:
   a. within 1 hour
   b. within 8 hours
   c. as long as 2 to 3 days
   d. as long as 4 to 5 days

5. Which of the following clients should not take a saline laxative?
   a. a 32-year-old diabetic
   b. a 55-year-old woman with breast cancer
   c. a 67-year-old male in congestive heart failure
   d. a 22-year-old who has AIDS

6. Which of the following laxatives would be used for rapid bowel movement?
   a. Metamucil
   b. Milk of magnesia
   c. Dulcolax
   d. castor oil

7. Your client is taking a bulk-forming laxative. Which of the following adverse effects will you observe for?
   a. fecal impaction
   b. diarrhea
   c. fluid retention
   d. edema

8. Which of the following drugs decrease the effects of laxatives and cathartics?
   a. Demerol
   b. Synthroid
   c. Inderal
   d. Dilantin

9. Instructions regarding administration of lactulose should include:
   a. Take with food.
   b. Take every other day.
   c. Take without food or liquid.
   d. Mix with fruit juice to improve taste.

10. The most abused laxative is a:
    a. surfactant laxative
    b. saline laxative
    c. stimulant cathartic
    d. lubricant laxative

CHAPTER 62

Antidiarrheals

■ Exercises

Match the following.

1. ____ loperamide (Imodium)

2. ____ nalaxone hydrochloride (Narcan)

3. ____ octreotide (Sandostatin)

4. ____ lactase deficiency

5. ____ ampicillin

6. ____ antibiotic-associated colitis

7. ____ diphenoxylate (Lomotil)

8. ____ cholestyramine (Questran)

9. ____ polycarbophil (FiberCon)

10. ____ gastroenteritis

11. ____ acute diarrhea

12. ____ tannin

13. ____ bismuth subalicylate (Pepto-Bismol)

14. ____ opiate derivatives

15. ____ chronic diarrhea

a. Mechanism by which the body tries to rid itself of irritants, toxins, and infectious agents

b. Occasionally used in diarrhea to decrease fluidity of stools

c. Inhibits digestion of milk and milk products, which causes diarrhea

d. Can cause malnutrition and anemia

e. Opiate derivative for diarrhea which requires a prescription

f. Used to treat diarrhea by binding and inactivating bile salts

g. May cause antibiotic-associated colitis

h. Used to treat diarrhea associated with carcinoid syndrome

i. Substance found in berry plants that reduces intestinal inflammation and secretions, and is used to treat diarrhea

j. A condition that can cause diarrhea

k. Associated with diarrhea containing mucus, pus, and blood

l. Antidote for overdose of loperamide (Imodium)

m. Most effective agents for symptomatic treatment of diarrhea

n. Over-the-counter bismuth salt

o. Nonprescription antidiarrheal drug

■ Clinical Challenge

A 68-year-old female alcoholic comes to the clinic complaining of diarrhea. She has had diarrhea for 2 weeks, and she is worried that something is wrong. A thorough assessment reveals that, about a month ago, she was constipated and took four different laxatives. Because all laboratory tests are negative, you suspect she is experiencing diarrhea from excessive use of laxatives. The physician prescribes diphenoxylate with atropine sulfate (Lomotil) PO 5 mg 3 to 4 times daily. Before the drug is started, what should the physician do? What should instructions for this client include? Identify two potential nursing diagnoses appropriate for this client.

▪ Review Questions

1. Your client, age 3, is admitted to the hospital with an overdose of loperamide (Imodium). Which of the following medications would be administered to him?

   a. meclizine hydrochloride (Antivert)

   b. naloxone (Narcan)

   c. diphenhydramine (Benadryl)

   d. hydroxyzine hydrochloride (Atarax)

2. A client is diagnosed with ulcerative colitis. Which of the following drugs would be prescribed for him?

   a. tacrine (Cognex)

   b. bethanechol (Urecholine)

   c. balsalazide (Colazal)

   d. furosemide (Lasix)

3. Your client experiences traveler's diarrhea. What should you suggest?

   a. colestipol (Colestid)

   b. psyllium preparation (Metamucil)

   c. loperamide (Imodium)

   d. bismuth subsalicylate (Pepto-Bismol)

4. A client develops diarrhea secondary to antibiotic therapy. He is to receive diphenoxylate (Lomotil) PO, 2 tablets PRN for each diarrheal stool. The nurse should inform him that he may experience:

   a. dizziness

   b. hypersensitivity reaction

   c. muscle aches

   d. increase in appetite

5. Your client has carcinoid syndrome. Which of the following drugs would he be taking for the diarrhea?

   a. loperamide (Imodium)

   b. octreotide (Sandostatin)

   c. difenoxin (Motofen)

   d. colestipol (Colestid)

6. The goal of drug therapy for diarrhea is to:

   a. prevent severe fluid and electrolyte loss

   b. increase weight by 2 to 5 pounds

   c. eliminate the bacterial organism

   d. decrease anal discomfort

7. Which of the following would be contraindicated in chronic diarrhea?

   a. antibacterial agents

   b. bismuth preparations

   c. psyllium preparations

   d. opiates

8. You are a home care nurse working with a client who has HIV/AIDS. The client has diarrhea and will be taking octreotide (Sandostatin). The client will self-administer the medication:

   a. by mouth

   b. subcutaneously

   c. in the deltoid muscle

   d. under the tongue

9. Instructions regarding the administration of paregoric should include:

   a. Add at least 30 mL of water to each dose.

   b. Take with 4 oz of water.

   c. Take after every meal.

   d. May include up to 8 doses daily.

10. Which of the following antidiarrheals is a nonprescription drug?

   a. loperamide (Imodium)

   b. diphenoxylate (Lomotil)

   c. difenoxin (Motofen)

   d. paregoric

CHAPTER 63

Antiemetics

■ Exercises

Fill in the blank.

1. The vomiting center is located in the _____ _____.

2. _____ and _____ are phenothiazines that are commonly used to prevent or treat nausea and vomiting.

3. _____ produce relaxation and inhibit the cerebral cortex.

4. _____ is a cannabinoid given to cancer patients to manage nausea and vomiting associated with chemotherapy.

5. _____ is used in the management of labyrinthitis.

6. An over-the-counter antiemetic given orally in 15-minute intervals is _____ _____.

7. _____ can be used as a transdermal patch to prevent seasickness.

8. _____ may increase the effects of alcohol and decrease the effects of digoxin.

9. The injectable form of _____ can be mixed in apple juice for clients who cannot swallow tablets.

10. A corticosteroid used in the management of chemotherapy-induced nausea and vomiting is _____.

Place a T (true) or F (false) in each blank.

1. ____ Most antiemetic drugs should be used cautiously in clients with liver disease.

2. ____ Older adults are usually more sensitive to dronabinol's psychoactive effects than younger adults.

3. ____ Nausea must occur prior to vomiting.

4. ____ All antihistamines are effective as antiemetics.

5. ____ Benzodiazepines are considered antiemetics.

6. ____ Phenothiazines act on the CTZ and the vomiting center to exert antiemetic effects.

7. ____ Dronabinol (Marinol) has a high potential for abuse.

8. ____ Metoclopramide (Reglan) is contraindicated in Parkinson's disease.

9. ____ The 5-HT3 receptor antagonists are the first choice for clients with chemotherapy-induced nausea and vomiting.

10. ____ Large doses of phenothiazines are needed to produce antiemetic effects.

■ Clinical Challenge

Your client is a 55-year-old female who is receiving chemotherapy for colon cancer. She is experiencing nausea and vomiting related to her treatments. Ondansetron (Zofran) has been prescribed for her. Why was this drug ordered for the client? List common adverse effects of ondansetron (Zofran).

The client continues to complain of nausea and vomiting. Which drug do you suspect the physician will add to the client's antiemetic regimen?

▪ Review Questions

1. A 50-year-old is receiving promethazine (Phenergan) for chemotherapy-induced emesis. The nurse will encourage:
   a. frequent oral care
   b. increased fluid intake
   c. a low-fat diet
   d. ambulation

2. A client is receiving metoclopramide (Reglan) for severe nausea. The nurse will monitor the client for which of the following adverse effects?
   a. hypoglycemia
   b. dystonia
   c. GERD
   d. photosensitivity

3. Your client has been on antiemetic therapy. Which of the following statements indicate a need for further instruction?
   a. "I should avoid driving my car while taking my medication."
   b. "If I start losing weight, I should let you know."
   c. "I enjoy drinking a glass of red wine every night."
   d. "I have stopped going to my exercise class since I have been on medication."

4. Your client is taking dronabinol (Marinol) for nausea and vomiting associated with chemotherapy. A possible concern for the client when the drug is discontinued is:
   a. urinary frequency
   b. sleep disturbance
   c. joint pain and stiffness
   d. decreased appetite

5. Which of the following clients would *not* be a candidate for metoclopramide (Reglan) therapy?
   a. a 65-year-old male with congestive heart failure
   b. a 42-year-old female with breast cancer
   c. a 33-year-old female with diabetic gastroparesis
   d. a 50-year-old male with esophageal reflux

6. Which of the following antiemetic drugs should not be given to a child under the age of 12?
   a. promethazine (Phenergan)
   b. ondansetron (Zofran)
   c. dronabinol (Marinol)
   d. scopolamine (Transderm Scop)

7. In older adults, a positive outcome of antiemetic therapy is:
   a. decrease in blood pressure
   b. weight gain of 2 pounds per week
   c. increased activity level
   d. electrolyte balance

8. Your client is taking an antiemetic. Which of the following nursing diagnoses would be appropriate for her?
   a. noncompliance: failure to take medication as prescribed
   b. injury: risk for
   c. disturbed sleep pattern
   d. inbalanced nutrition, more than body requirements

9. A 28-year-old female is in the clinic for antiemetic therapy. She is going on an ocean cruise and expects to experience motion sickness. Instructions regarding this medication will include:
   a. Take medication at first sign of nausea.
   b. Take 30 minutes prior to getting on the ship and then every 4 to 6 hours as needed.
   c. Take medication with food.
   d. Take 10 minutes before getting on the ship, then once a day throughout the cruise.

10. A client, age 40, is receiving chemotherapy for ovarian cancer. To decrease the adverse effects of the chemotherapy, the nurse will administer metoclopramide (Reglan):

   a. immediately after the chemotherapy treatment

   b. every 4 hours PO during the treatment

   c. IV 30 to 60 minutes prior to the chemotherapy treatment

   d. IM just prior to chemotherapy treatment

CHAPTER 64

Drugs Used in Oncologic Disorders

■ Exercises

Place a T (true) or F (false) in each blank.

1. ____ For most cancers, it may take years to produce a detectable tumor.

2. ____ Leukemias are cancers of lymphoid tissues.

3. ____ Chemotherapy is the treatment of choice for colon cancer.

4. ____ Antineoplastic drugs are sometimes used to treat rheumatoid arthritis.

5. ____ Alkylating agents cause significant myelosuppression.

6. ____ Taxanes are used for early stages of breast and ovarian cancers.

7. ____ Cytotoxic chemotherapy is most effective when started before extensive tumor growth.

8. ____ Most chemotherapy regimens use single-drug therapy.

9. ____ Antineoplastic drugs are usually given in low doses on a cyclic schedule.

10. ____ Normal cells repair themselves faster than malignant cells.

Match the following drugs with the disease process for which they are used.

1. ____ etoposide (VePesid)

2. ____ topetecan (Hycamtin)

3. ____ doxorubicin liposomal (Doxil)

4. ____ cisplatin (Platinol)

5. ____ bleomycin (Blenoxane)

6. ____ methotrexate (Mexate)

7. ____ 5-fluorouracil (5-FU)

8. ____ cyclophosphamide (Cytoxan)

9. ____ vincristine (Oncovin)

10. ____ tamoxifen (Nolvadex)

a. Leukemias

b. Squamous cell carcinoma

c. Colon cancer

d. Small-cell lung cancer, advanced ovarian cancer

e. Wilms' tumor, neuroblastoma

f. Hodgkin's disease

g. AIDs-related Kaposi's sarcoma

h. Advanced carcinomas of testes, bladder, ovary

i. Prophylaxis and treatment of metastatic breast cancer

j. Testicular cancer

■ Clinical Challenge

Your client is a 49-year-old female diagnosed with ovarian cancer. She is to begin chemotherapy with doxorubicin (Adriamycin) and cyclosphosphamide (Cytoxan). Why does her treatment regimen include two antineoplastic agents? Describe the adverse effects she is likely to experience with these drugs.

After 3 weeks, your client has lost all of her hair. She is depressed and withdrawn. How will you intervene?

■ Review Questions

1. Your client is being treated with fluorouracil (5-FU) for breast cancer. Your teaching plan will include:

    a. increase in activity

    b. avoidance of fat in the diet

    c. frequent oral hygiene

    d. restriction of fluid intake

2. A 52-year-old female is taking tamoxifen (Nolvadex). Which of the following will need monitoring during therapy?

    a. creatinine level

    b. liver enzymes

    c. blood glucose

    d. weight

3. Hospitalization is recommended for the first course of treatment for which of the following drugs?

    a. melphalan

    b. procarbazine

    c. bleomycine

    d. gencitabine

4. Which of the following should be evaluated before and during methotrexate (Mexate) therapy?

    a. visual acuity

    b. blood pressure

    c. hepatic function

    d. renal status

5. A client is receiving vincristine (Oncovin) intravenously weekly. He may experience:

    a. severe headache

    b. tingling of the arms and legs

    c. dry mouth

    d. irritability

6. An adverse effect of cisplatin (Platinol) is:

    a. ototoxicity

    b. diarrhea

    c. bleeding gums

    d. mucositis

7. Your client is a 28-year-old diagnosed with Hodgkin's disease. He is receiving vincristine (Oncovin) therapy. When planning care for your client, you will plan to:

    a. monitor blood glucose levels

    b. limit solid foods throughout therapy

    c. sedate him during the infusions

    d. observe for IV infiltration

8. A client is taking oral cyclophosphamide (Cytoxan) therapy. Because hemorrhagic urethritis is an adverse effect, you will encourage:

    a. drinking lots of fluids

    b. limiting fluid intake

    c. taking the medication at bedtime

    d. increasing protein in the diet

9. When taking methotrexate (Mexate), a client should avoid:

    a. Tylenol

    b. vitamin K

    c. aspirin

    d. sodium

10. To prevent thrombocytopenia as a result of chemotherapy, a client may be given:

    a. mesna (Mesnex)

    b. amifostine (Ethyol)

    c. dexrazoxane (Zinecard)

    d. oprelvekin (Neumega)

■Cell Cycle Diagram

In spaces 1–5 provided in Figure 64-1, explain what happens during each phase of cell replication. On lines a–h, identify the antineoplastic agents that are effective in each phase.

Antibiotics   Antimetabolites
Alkylating agents   Steroids
Podophyllotoxins   Taxanes or taxoids
Nitrosoureas   Vinca alkaloids

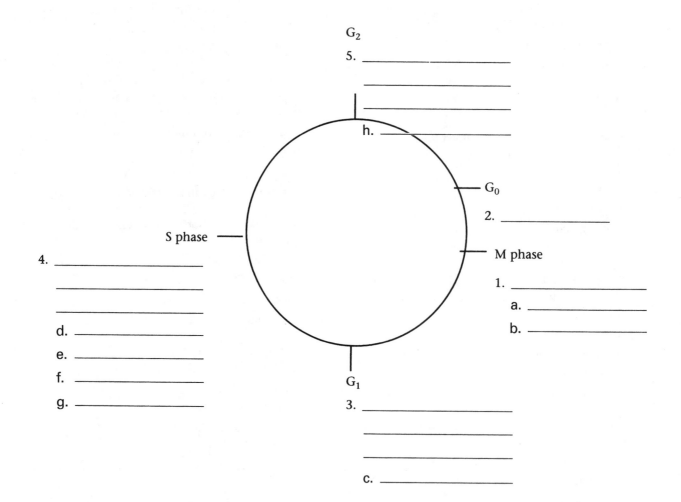

FIGURE 64-1.

CHAPTER 65

Drugs Used in Ophthalmic Conditions

■ Exercises

Match the following.

1. ____ conjunctiva
2. ____ hyperopia
3. ____ miosis
4. ____ aqueous humor
5. ____ keratitis
6. ____ blepharitis
7. ____ glaucoma
8. ____ myopia
9. ____ conjunctivitis
10. ____ mydriasis

a. The mucous membrane lining of the eyelids
b. Inflammation of the cornea
c. Nearsightedness
d. Chronic infection of glands and lash follicles in the margins of the eyelids
e. Pupil constriction
f. Common eye disorder characterized by redness, tearing, itching, edema, and a burning sensation
g. Farsightedness
h. Pupil dilation
i. Clear fluid produced by capillaries in the ciliary body
j. Disease characterized by optic nerve damage, changes in visual fields, and increased intraocular pressure

Place a T (true) or F (false) in each blank.

1. ____ Eye ointments should be administered more often than eye drops.

2. ____ Systemic administration is the most common route for ophthalmic drugs.

3. ____ When administering multiple eye drops, there should be intervals of 5 to 10 minutes between applications.

4. ____ Topical ophthalmic medications should be discarded after the expiration date.

5. ____ Topical ophthalmic medications can be safely applied while wearing soft contact lenses.

6. ____ Ocular infections are often treated with broad-spectrum antibacterial agents.

7. ____ Nonprescription eye drops should never be used longer than 72 hours.

8. ____ Most ophthalmic drops contain sulfites, which can cause allergic reactions.

9. ____ Normal intraocular pressure is less than 12 mm Hg.

10. ____ Glaucoma is a common, preventable cause of blindness.

Fill in the blank.

1. The _____ _____ refracts light rays and helps maintain the normal shape of the eyeball.

2. The innermost layer of the eyeball is the _____.

3. The area where the optic nerve and blood vessels enter the eyeball is called the _____ _____.

4. _____ is the drug of choice for eye infections caused by the herpes simplex virus.

5. _____ is the drug of choice in fungal eye infections.

6. _____ _____ _____ are first-choice drugs used in chronic glaucoma.

7. Older adults are at high risk for _____ and _____.

8. For ophthalmoscopic examinations in children, _____ and _____ are preferred.

9. Long-term use of corticosteroids can raise intraocular pressure and cause _____.

10. With _____ _____, permanent darkening of eye color may occur.

■ Clinical Challenge

A 58-year-old housewife is in for a routine eye exam. She has no complaints and states that she has had no problems with her glasses. The examination reveals a significant increase in intraocular pressure from last year. Past examinations have noted a steady increase in the past 3 years. The physician orders pilocarpine (Pilocar). Why was this medication ordered for her? How do you instruct the client to administer the drops?

The client asks you how long she will have to use the medication. How do you respond?

■ Review Questions

1. Your client has recently been diagnosed with open-angle glaucoma. She is to begin treatment with pilocarpine (Pilocar) 0.25%, 2 gtt every 6 hours. You will caution her that the most common adverse effects are:
   a. irritability and mood swings
   b. increased pulse and heart palpitations
   c. itching and burning
   d. anorexia and weight loss

2. A 48-year-old client is to begin timolol maleate (Timoptic) 1 gt OS twice a day. Prior to beginning therapy, the nurse will evaluate the client for:
   a. diabetes mellitus
   b. renal impairment
   c. liver disease
   d. respiratory and cardiac problems

3. While administering a mydriatic into your client's eyes, he asks you how long it will take for the pupils to dilate. Your response should be:
   a. "Not long."
   b. "About 30 minutes."
   c. "Between 5 and 15 minutes."
   d. "No longer than a couple of minutes."

4. When assessing a client's eyes after the administration of pilocarpine (Pilocar), the nurse will anticipate:
   a. dilated pupils
   b. constricted pupils
   c. increased visual acuity
   d. decrease in aqueous humor

5. A diagnosis of conjunctivitis is made for your client. Gentamicin (Garamycin) 1 drop every 4 hours in both eyes is prescribed. It would be important for you to determine whether he has a history of:
   a. drug abuse
   b. allergic reactions
   c. diabetes mellitus
   d. mental illness

6. Before the administration of eye drops, the nurse's initial action should be to:

   a. warm the medication

   b. take the blood pressure

   c. ask the client to lie down

   d. wash his or her hands

7. After the administration of a miotic drug in both eyes, a client may complain of:

   a. halos around lights

   b. decreased vision in dim light

   c. pain in both eyes

   d. nausea and vomiting

8. Systemic absorption from ophthalmic administration can be prevented by:

   a. applying pressure to the inner canthus after administration of the medication

   b. administering the drug at bedtime

   c. placing a warm, moist towel over the eyes after administration of the medication

   d. rinsing the eyes with sterile water after administering the medication

9. Your client is taking a prostaglandin analog for glaucoma. You suspect which of the following adverse effects?

   a. nausea and vomiting

   b. dehydration

   c. upper respiratory and flu-like symptoms

   d. dry mouth

10. Which of the following drugs would be indicated for ocular itching due to seasonal allergies?

    a. diclofenac (Voltaren)

    b. flurbiprofen (Ocufen)

    c. ketorolac (Acular)

    d. suprofen (Profenal)

■ Anatomy of the Eye Diagram

Fill in the blanks in Figure 65-1 with the terms below.

Iris	Pupil	Sclera
Cornea	Anterior changer	Optic nerve
Lens	Retina	Optic disc
Vitreous body	Choroid	

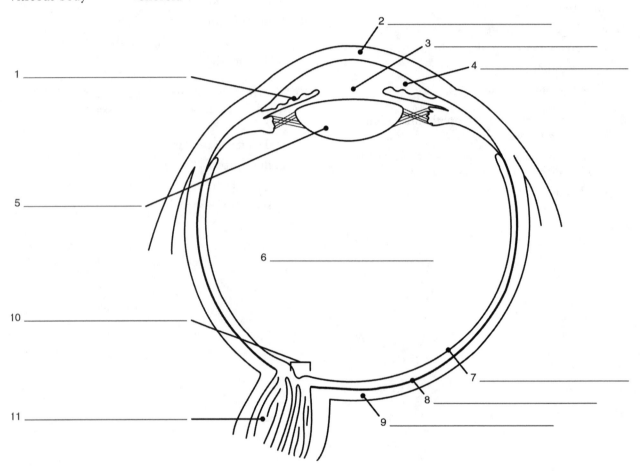

FIGURE 65-1.

CHAPTER 66

Drugs Used in Dermatologic Conditions

■ Exercises

Match the following.

1. _____ psoriasis

2. _____ folliculitis

3. _____ *Candida albicans*

4. _____ cellulitis

5. _____ furuncles

6. _____ astringent

7. _____ impetigo

8. _____ retinoids

9. _____ aloe

10. _____ dermatitis

11. _____ oral candidiasis

12. _____ benzoyl peroxide

13. _____ urticaria

14. _____ keratolytic agents

15. _____ rosacea

a. Characterized by erythema; flushing; fine, red superficial blood vessels, and acne-like lesions of the face

b. Infection of the hair follicles that occurs on the scalp or bearded areas of the face

c. Fungal infection that usually occurs after the use of a broad-spectrum systemic antibiotic

d. Vitamin A derivatives used to treat acne, psoriasis, aging, and wrinkling of the skin

e. Skin lesions called wheals, "hives"

f. Characterized by erythema, tenderness, edema with malaise, chills, and fever

g. Causes most fungal infections of the skin

h. "Boils"

i. Skin disorder characterized by erythematous, dry, scaling lesions

j. Topical substance used for minor burns and wounds

k. Superficial skin infection caused by streptococci or staphylococci

l. An inflammatory response of the skin to injuries

m. Used to remove warts, corns, and calluses

n. A topical bactericidal agent

o. Drying agent

Place a T (true) or F (false) in each blank.

1. _____ The skin is the smallest organ of the body.

2. _____ The skin's pH is acidic.

3. _____ Scratching can damage skin and cause secondary infections.

4. _____ Hyperplasia of the nose (rhinophyma) can develop from intertrigo.

5. _____ Tinea capitis is the most common type of ringworm infection.

6. _____ Increased secretion of androgens at puberty in both sexes may contribute to acne

7. _____ Chocolate and fatty foods increase the severity of acne.

8. _____ External otitis is most often caused by beta-hemolytic streptococci.

9. _____ Tacrolimus (Protopic) ointment can be used in children as young as 2 years of age.

10. _____ Most dermatologic medications are applied topically.

■ Clinical Challenge

Your client is a 20-year-old female who comes to the clinic with severe cystic acne. She has been followed by her hometown physician, who treated her with tetracycline and benzoyl peroxide without much success. Isotretinoin (Accutane) is prescribed for her. Why was this drug prescribed for the client? What special instructions should you give to the client? How long do you suspect she will take Accutane?

■ Review Questions

1. Before topical application of a medication, the nurse should:

    a. rinse the area with cold water

    b. scrub the skin area and rub dry

    c. expose skin area to a heat lamp

    d. wash the skin and pat dry

2. Your client has been taking isotretinoin (Accutane) for 2 months. You will assess for which of the following during a follow-up clinic visit?

    a. increased blood pressure

    b. depression

    c. irritability

    d. dry mouth

3. Your 16-year-old client has started taking an oral retinoid. She should avoid:

    a. dairy products

    b. carbonated drinks

    c. extremely cold air

    d. vitamin A supplements

4. A client is taking an oral antihistamine to relieve itching associated with a contact dermatitis. Instructions should include:

    a. "Take oral medication on a regular schedule, around the clock."

    b. "Take only when itching is worse."

    c. "Use in combination with a topical medication to decrease itching."

    d. "You may increase dosage as itching severity warrants."

5. A 22-year-old female has been diagnosed with acne vulgaris. Tetracycline has been ordered. Which of the following would be an appropriate question to ask her before therapy is started?

    a. "How long have you had the cyst-like nodules in your face?"

    b. "When was your last menstrual period?"

    c. "How many times a day do you scrub your face?"

    d. "Have you been taking any oral medication for the acne?"

6. You are caring for a 28-year-old male who has second-degree burns on his hands and arms. Treatment includes application of silver sulfadiazine (Silvadene) to the burn area twice a day. Intervention should include:

    a. washing area with warm water before application of Silvadene

    b. applying salve after Silvadene to seal medication over skin area

    c. applying the medication using sterile technique

    d. applying the medication at bedtime

7. A client has used a topical corticosteroid for several days to treat psoriasis. Which of the following adverse effects may occur?

    a. increase in blood pressure

    b. atrophy of the skin

    c. anorexia

    d. burning sensation in area of application

8. Chronic dry or scaly lesions are best treated with:

    a. aerosol sprays

    b. gels

    c. ointments

    d. lotions

9. Your client, a 15-year-old male, is beginning drug therapy for acne. Instructions concerning benzoyl peroxide should include:

   a. Overuse can cause extreme dryness of skin.

   b. Use caution when driving or operating machinery.

   c. Adverse effects are nausea and vomiting.

   d. A decrease in appetite may occur.

10. Systemic effects of clobetasol (Temovate) include:

    a. hypotension

    b. suppression of adrenal function

    c. muscle spasms

    d. stimulation of hepatic enzymes

CHAPTER 67

Drugs Used During Pregnancy and Lactation

■ Exercises

Place a T (true) or F (false) in each blank.

1. _____ Many drugs are considered safe during pregnancy.

2. _____ Drug effects are more predictable during pregnancy than when in the nonpregnant state.

3. _____ In the fetus, a large proportion of a drug dose is active because the fetus has low levels of serum albumin and low levels of drug binding.

4. _____ Drug teratogenicity is most likely to occur during the first trimester of pregnancy.

5. _____ Small amounts of alcohol during pregnancy are considered safe.

6. _____ Caffeine is the most commonly ingested drug during pregnancy.

7. _____ Cigarette smoking during pregnancy can cause fetal and infant death.

8. _____ Marijuana can cause third-trimester bleeding.

9. _____ Abruptio placentae can occur from ingestion of cocaine during the third semester of pregnancy.

10. _____ Herbal supplements are recommended during pregnancy.

11. _____ Human insulin may be needed during gestational diabetes.

12. _____ Amoxicillin may be used to treat a urinary tract infection during pregnancy.

13. _____ Women who are insulin dependent are more likely to need smaller doses during pregnancy.

14. _____ Clonidine is the drug of choice for the pregnant hypertensive woman.

15. _____ Women with epilepsy should double their routine dose of folic acid during pregnancy.

Match the following.

1. _____ ferrous sulfate

2. _____ magnesium sulfate

3. _____ meclizine (Antivert)

4. _____ aspirin

5. _____ ritodrine (Yutopar)

6. _____ oxytocin (Pitocin)

7. _____ folic acid

8. _____ methylergonovine (Methergine)

9. _____ meperidine (Demerol)

10. _____ Metamucil

a. Used to treat anemia during pregnancy

b. May be used for prophylaxis in women at risk of developing preeclampsia

c. Used to treat nausea and vomiting during pregnancy

d. Drug of choice used to prevent or treat seizures during preeclampsia and eclampsia

e. Stimulates uterine contractions to initiate labor

f. Opioid analgesic used during labor and delivery

g. May be used during pregnancy for constipation

h. Used in the management of postpartum hemorrhage

i. Relaxes uterine smooth muscle, which will slow or stop uterine contractions

j. Necessary to prevent neural tube birth defects

■ Clinical Challenge

Your client is a 28-year-old who is 30 weeks pregnant and has diabetes mellitus. She is insulin dependent and is being followed closely by a home health nurse. The client presents with signs of preterm labor in the emergency department. She is admitted and started on IV ritodrine (Yutopar). How will you prepare ritodrine for administration? How long will the client receive this medication?

In order to facilitate uterine placental blood flow, how should the client be positioned during the administration of the medication?

Uterine suppression is successful, and the client is to be discharged on an oral dosage of ritodrine. What instructions do you give to the client?

■ Review Questions

1. Your client is 20 weeks pregnant, and fetal heart tones can no longer be heard. It is determined that the pregnancy is to be terminated. Which of the following drugs will be given after mifepristone to make sure of full expulsion of the conceptus?

   a. ritodrine

   b. prostaglandin

   c. methylergonovine

   d. oxytocin

2. Your client is receiving a tocolytic. Which of the following may indicate hypermagnesemia?

   a. increased blood pressure of 170/90

   b. decreased heart rate of 60

   c. decreased respiratory rate of 8

   d. increased body temperature of 102°

3. Which of the following indicates an appropriate dose of vitamin K for a neonate at delivery?

   a. 0.25 to 0.5 mg

   b. 0.5 to 1 mg

   c. 1 to 1.5 mg

   d. 2.5 to 5 mg

4. You are counseling a group of pregnant women at the health department concerning use of immunizations during pregnancy. You should stress that which of the following immunizations should not be taken during pregnancy?

   a. influenza

   b. rubella

   c. hepatitis B

   d. tetanus

5. Oxytocin is the drug of choice for prevention and control of postpartum uterine hemorrhage because it is unlikely to cause:

   a. hypotension

   b. hypertension

   c. tachycardia

   d. bradycardia

6. A new mother who is breastfeeding questions you concerning use of antihistamines for her allergies. An appropriate response would be:

   a. "An antihistamine may cause you to be drowsy."

   b. "As long as you take only one a day, it should be all right."

   c. "Antihistamines can cause a decrease in milk production."

   d. "Antihistamines may cause your baby's heart rate to increase."

7. Which of the following drugs should be completely avoided during pregnancy?

   a. nicotine

   b. caffeine

   c. acetaminophen

   d. alcohol

8. Tetracyclines are contraindicated during pregnancy because they:

   a. decrease the white blood cell count in the mother

   b. interfere with the development of teeth and bone in the fetus

   c. interfere with folic acid metabolism in the fetus

   d. cause long bone growth retardation in the fetus

9. A 40-year-old has just been told she is pregnant by her health care provider. She has a history of mild hypertension and is concerned about taking medication during pregnancy. An appropriate response should include:

   a. "Hydralazine is considered safe to use during pregnancy."

   b. "Guanfacine can be used in reduced dosages."

   c. "All antihypertensive drugs are unsafe to use during pregnancy."

   d. "Clonidine can be used."

10. Which of the following drugs is used to promote fetal production of surfactant?

    a. furosemide

    b. ergotamine

    c. nifedipine

    d. betamethasone

Answers

Chapter 1

DEFINITIONS

pharmacology—the study of drugs that alter functions of living organisms

biotechnology—involves manipulation of DNA and RNA in the development of drugs

drug therapy—the use of drugs to prevent, diagnose, or cure disease processes or to relieve signs and symptoms

prototypes—individual drugs that represent a group of drugs

medications—drugs that are given for therapeutic purposes

generic drug name—derived from the chemical or official name and is independent of a manufacturer

systemic drug effects—those resulting from drugs are absorbed into the bloodstream and circulated through the body

trade drug name—name given to a drug and patented by the manufacturer

synthetic chemical compounds—drugs manufactured in laboratories

over-the-counter (OTC)—refers to drugs that can be purchased without a prescription

SHORT ANSWER

1. Synthetic drugs are more standardized in chemical characteristics, more consistent in effects, and less likely to produce allergic reactions
2. Involves the costs of drug therapy, including purchasing, dispensing, storage, administration, laboratory, and other tests used to monitor client responses and losses from expiration
3. By prescription or order from licensed health care provider and by over-the-counter purchase of drugs that do not require a prescription
4. Trade names are capitalized; generic names are lowercase
5. According to their effects on certain body systems, their therapeutic uses, and chemical characteristics

FILL IN THE CHART

Name	Year	Provision
Comprehensive Drug Abuse Prevention and Control Act	1970	Regulated distribution of narcotics and other drugs of abuse
Durham-Humphrey	1952	Designated drugs that are prescribed by a physician and dispensed by a pharmacist
Kefauver-Harris Amendment	1962	Required proof that drugs were effective for how they were labeled
Harrison Narcotic Act	1914	Controlled the manufacture, importation, transportation, and distribution of opium, cocaine, marijuana, and their derivatives
Sherley Amendment	1912	Prohibited fraudulent claims of efficacy

MATCHING

1. e   2. a   3. b   4. d   5. c   6. b   7. a   8. d
9. e   10. d

REVIEW QUESTIONS

1. b   2. a   3. c   4. d   5. b   6. c   7. b   8. c
9. d   10. a

CELL PHYSIOLOGY DIAGRAM, PART I

1. Cell membrane
2. Cytoplasm
3. Lysosomes
4. Nucleus
5. Chromatin
6. Endoplasmic reticulum
7. Ribosomes
8. Golgi apparatus
9. Mitochondria

CELL PHYSIOLOGY DIAGRAM, PART II
1. Drug movement and therefore drug action are affected by a drug's ability to cross cell membranes.
2. Prostaglandins and histamine are released in response to cellular damage and cause vasodilation, vascular permeability, pain, and edema.

Chapter 2

MATCHING
1. c   2. i   3. d   4. k   5. e   6. f   7. l   8. m
9. o   10. g   11. a   12. h   13. n   14. j   15. b

SHORT ANSWER
1. Age, body weight, genetic and ethnic characteristics, gender, pathologic conditions, psychological considerations
2. Allergic reactions, damaging body tissues, increasing body heat, interference with dissipation of body heat, action on the temperature regulating center in the brain
3. Supporting and stabilizing vital functions, preventing further damage from the toxic agent, administering specific antidotes
4. Water, electrolytes, proteins, lipids, carbohydrates
5. Direct penetration, protein channels, carrier proteins

DEFINITIONS
1. Involves drug movement from an area of higher concentration to one of lower concentration
2. Similar to passive diffusion except drug molecules combine with a carrier protein or enzyme
3. Drug molecules move from an area of lower concentration to one of higher concentration; requires a carrier substance and release of cellular energy

FILL IN THE CHART

Drug	Antidote
heparin	protamine sulfate
opioid analgesics	naloxone (Narcan)
phenothiazine	diphenhydramine (Benadryl)
warfarin (Coumadin)	vitamin K
acetaminophen	acetylcysteine (Mucomyst)
beta blockers	glucagon

REVIEW QUESTIONS
1. c   2. b   3. d   4. c   5. d   6. c   7. a   8. c
9. a   10. a

Chapter 3

DEFINITIONS
1. Right drug, dose, client, route, and time
2. The nurse is liable for his/her actions and is expected to have knowledge concerning all medications he/she is responsible for administering.
3. Name of client; generic or trade name of the drug; the dose, the route and frequency of administration; and the date, time, and signature of the prescriber
4. Any route other than gastrointestinal—denotes SC, IM, and IV
5. Because they contain high amounts of a drug intended to be absorbed slowly and act over an extended period of time

TRUE OR FALSE
1. f   2. t   3. f   4. f   5. f   6. t   7. t   8. t
9. f   10. t   11. f   12. f   13. t   14. f   15. t

MATCHING
1. g   2. m   3. j   4. e   5. o   6. i   7. b   8. c
9. d   10. f   11. a   12. k   13. l   14. h   15. n

FILL IN THE BLANK
1. 2.2   2. 1000   3. 1   4. 1   5. 15 or 16
6. 250   7. 1000   8. 1   9. 4 or 5   10. 1

FILL IN THE BLANK
1. 30   2. 22.73   3. 8 or 10
4. 3.5   5. 10 or 12.5 6. 15
7. 2000   8. 2   9. 2
10. 2500

CALCULATING DRUG DOSAGES
1. 4 tablets
2. 10 mL
3. 60 mL
4. 1.5 mL
5. 2 tablets
6. 11.25 mL
7. 2 capsules
8. 0.5 mL
9. 2 mL
10. 15 cc

REVIEW QUESTIONS
1. b   2. c   3. d   4. b   5. d   6. d   7. d   8. d
9. a   10. a

SUBCUTANEOUS INJECTIONS DIAGRAM 3-1

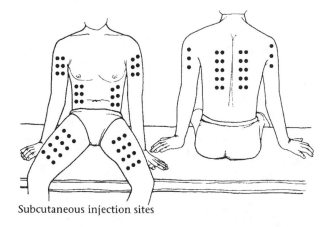

Subcutaneous injection sites

Chapter 4

FILL IN THE BLANK
1. nursing process
2. assessment
3. client
4. outcomes
5. critical paths

SHORT ANSWER
1. Deficient knowledge: drug therapy regimen; deficient knowledge: safe and effective self-administration; risk for injury related to adverse drug effects; noncompliance: overuse; noncompliance: underuse
2. Take drugs as prescribed; experience relief of s/s; accurately self-administer a drug; report use of herbal and dietary supplements
3. Assessment, drug administration, teaching, solving problems related to drug therapy, promoting compliance with prescribed drug therapy and identifying barriers to compliance, identifying resources for obtaining medication
4. Promoting healthy lifestyles, exercise, rest, sleep, handwashing, positioning, assisting with cough and deep breathing, ambulating, heat and cold
5. Because most medications are self administered and clients need information and assistance to use drugs safely and effectively.
6. Emphasis on outpatient treatments, short hospitalization period, client's reluctance to admit to noncompliance
7. Medical diagnosis, aspects of care related to medical diagnosis, desired client outcomes, and time frames for desired outcomes
8. The 1994 Dietary Supplement Health and Education Act (DSHEA) defined a dietary supplement as "a vitamin, a mineral, an herb, or other botanical used to supplement the diet." Herbs can be labeled according to their possible effects on the body but are not used to diagnose, prevent, relieve, or cure diseases unless approved by the FDA.

9. Use of supplements may keep the client from seeking treatment from a health care provider when indicated, and the products may interact with prescription drugs to decrease therapeutic effects or increase adverse effects.
10. Child's weight, age, and level of growth and development

TRUE OR FALSE
1. f   2. t   3. f   4. t   5. t   6. f   7. t   8. f
9. t   10. t   11. t   12. f   13. t   14. t   15. f

MATCHING
1. e   2. m   3. l   4. f   5. j   6. h   7. b   8. g
9. b   10. a   11. d   12. i   13. c   14. c and k   15. k

REVIEW QUESTIONS
1. d   2. d   3. b   4. b   5. b   6. a   7. c   8. d
9. b   10. b

Chapter 5

MATCHING
1. f   2. a   3. i   4. g   5. c   6. h   7. d   8. j
9. e   10. b

FILL IN THE BLANK
1. depressants, stimulants
2. spinal cord
3. glia, neuron
4. amino acids, amines, peptides
5. calcium ions
6. cell body, dendrite, axon
7. electrical, chemical
8. axon
9. norepinephrine
10. thalamus

SHORT ANSWER
1. Drowsiness, sleep, decreased muscle tone, decreased ability to move, and decreased perception of sensations
2. Wakefulness, decreased fatigue, mental alertness, hyperactivity, excessive talking, nervousness, and insomnia
3. The ability to produce an action potential or be stimulated (excitability) and the ability to convey electrical impulses (conductivity)
4. Transportation back into the presynaptic nerve terminal for reuse; diffusion into surrounding body fluids; destruction by enzymes
5. Availability of precursor proteins and enzymes required to synthesize neurotransmitters; the number and binding capacity of receptors in the cell membranes of pre- and postsynaptic nerve endings; acid-base imbalances; drugs

REVIEW QUESTIONS
1. d   2. a   3. a   4. c   5. b   6. a   7. c   8. d
9. b   10. a

NEUROTRANSMISSION DIAGRAM, PART I
1. Synapse
2. Release site
3. Postsynaptic nerve terminal
4. Receptor sites
5. Postsynaptic nerve cell membrane
6. Presynaptic nerve cell membrane
7. Neurotransmitters
8. Presynaptic nerve terminal

NEUROTRANSMISSION DIAGRAM, PART II
1. Synapse, receptors
2. Receptor sites

Chapter 6

MATCHING
1. d   2. j   3. h   4. b   5. g   6. c   7. a   8. e
9. f   10 i

SHORT ANSWER
1. The signal from nociceptors in peripheral tissues must be transmitted to the spinal cord, then to the hypothalamus and cerebral cortex in the brain.
2. According to point of origin in body structures (somatic, visceral, or neuropathic), duration (acute or chronic), or cause
3. Binds with opioid receptor to relieve pain by inhibiting the release of substance P in central and peripheral nerves, decreasing the perception of pain sensation in the brain
4. Analgesia, drowsiness to sleep to unconsciousness, decreased mental and physical activity, respiratory depression, nausea and vomiting, and pupil constriction
5. Further depress respirations
6. Agonists—include morphine and morphine-like drugs; produce prototypical opioid effects. Antagonists— antidote drugs that reverse the effects of opioid agonists. However, the drugs can have agonistic activity at some receptors and antagonistic activity at other receptors.
7. Reverse or block analgesia, CNS respiratory depression, compete with opioids at opioid receptors
8. There is no upper limit to the dosage that can be given to clients who have developed tolerance to previous dosages.
9. Oral doses go through extensive metabolism on their first pass through the liver.
10. Aggressiveness, restlessness, body aches, insomnia, piloerection, nausea and vomiting, diarrhea, increased body temperature, increased respiratory rate and blood pressure, abdominal and muscle cramps, dehydration, and weight loss

TRUE OR FALSE
1. f   2. t   3. f   4. t   5. t   6. f   7. f   8. t
9. t   10. t

REVIEW QUESTIONS
1. b   2. b   3. d   4. d   5. a   6. b   7. b   8. a
9. a   10. b

Chapter 7

MATCHING
1. i   2. c   3. e   4. d   5. f   6. g   7. h   8. j
9. a   10. b

TRUE OR FALSE
1. f   2. t   3. f   4. t   5. t   6. f   7. t   8. t
9. f   10. t

MATCHING
1. h   2. e   3. j   4. f   5. i   6. g   7. c   8. d
9. a   10. b

REVIEW QUESTIONS
1. a   2. b   3. c   4. d   5. d   6. b   7. b   8. d
9. b   10. b

Chapter 8

MATCHING
1. h   2. j   3. a   4. i   5. d   6. e   7. b   8. f
9. c   10. g

SHORT ANSWER
1. Does not cause drowsiness
2. Highly lipid-soluble, allows drugs to enter CNS and perform their actions. Drugs redistributed to peripheral tissues, then slowly eliminated
3. Severe respiratory disease, severe liver or kidney disease, hypersensitivity reactions, history of alcohol and other drug abuse
4. Buspirone lacks muscle relaxant and anticonvulsant effects, does not cause sedation or physical or psychological dependence, does not increase CNS depression of alcohol and other drugs, and is not a controlled substance
5. To relieve anxiety or sleeplessness without permitting sensory perception, responsiveness to the environment, or alertness to drop below safe levels

FILL IN THE BLANK
1. chlordiazepoxide
2. zolpidem
3. midazolam
4. buspirone
5. hydroxyzine
6. alprazolam

7. zaleplon
8. sertraline
9. lorazepam
10. temazepam

TRUE OR FALSE
1. t   2. f   3. f   4. t   5. t   6. f   7. t   8. t
9. t   10. t

REVIEW QUESTIONS
1. c   2. d   3. a   4. b   5. a   6. c   7. a   8. b
9. a   10. b

Chapter 9

TRUE OR FALSE
1. f   2. t   3. t   4. t   5. f   6. t   7. f   8. t
9. f   10. t

SHORT ANSWER
1. Agitation, behavioral disturbances, delusions, disorganized speech, hallucinations, insomnia, and paranoia
2. Lack of pleasure, motivation, a blunted affect, poor grooming and hygiene, poor social skills, poor speech, and social withdrawal
3. Typical—older, have more adverse effects, act mainly on positive symptoms of schizophrenia
   Atypical—newer, fewer adverse effects, act on both positive and negative symptoms of schizophrenia
4. Nausea, vomiting, and intractable hiccups
5. Causes agranulocytosis, a life-threatening blood disease, occurs in first 3 weeks of therapy

FILL IN THE BLANK
1. clozapine
2. dopamine
3. schizophrenia
4. haloperidol
5. pimozide
6. clozapine
7. promethazine
8. thioridazine
9. extrapyramidal effects
10. jaundice

REVIEW QUESTIONS
1. b   2. a   3. c   4. d   5. d   6. a   7. c   8. b
9. c   10. a

Chapter 10

SHORT ANSWER
1. Depression thought to result from deficiency of norepinephrine and or serotonin. Thought that

antidepressant drugs increase amounts of one or both of these in the CNS synapse.
2. Corticotropin-releasing factor increased in depression, which leads to increase in cortisol, which leads to decrease in cortisol receptors, which leads to depression. Also, abnormalities in secretion of thyroid and growth hormones can lead to depression.
3. Immune system; genetic factors; environmental factors
4. Tricyclics (TCAs); monoamine oxidase inhibitors (MAOIs); selective serotonin reuptake inhibitors (SSRIs)
5. Normalizes abnormal neurotransmission systems in the brain by altering the amounts of neurotransmitters and number of receptors
6. Aged cheese and meats; concentrated yeast extracts; sauerkraut; fava beans
7. Client's age; medical condition; history of drug response; drug adverse effects
8. Are effective and produce fewer and milder adverse effects
9. To prevent suicide
10. Occurs 1 to 4 hours after drug ingestion, causes nystagmus, tremors, restlessness, seizures, hypotension, dysrhythmias, myocardial depression

FILL IN THE BLANK
1. 2.5
2. bupropion
3. depression
4. hyperglycemia
5. hyperthermia
6. receptors
7. MAOIs,
8. fluoxetine
9. lithium
10. St. John's wort

FILL IN THE CHART
TCAs—sedation, orthostatic hypotension, cardiac dysrhythmias, blurred vision, dry mouth, constipation, urinary retention, weight gain, sexual dysfunction

SSRIs—nausea, diarrhea, weight loss, sexual dysfunction, anxiety, nervousness, insomnia

MAOIs—severe hypertension, blurred vision, constipation, dizziness, dry mouth, hypotension, urinary retention, hypoglycemia

MATCHING
1. f   2. j   3. e   4. b   5. a   6. h   7. d   8. i
9. g   10. c

REVIEW QUESTIONS
1. c   2. c   3. c   4. b   5. b   6. c   7. d   8. a
9. c   10. b

Chapter 11

MATCHING
1. g   2. j   3. i   4. b   5. h   6. e   7. a   8. f
9. d   10. c

FILL IN THE BLANK
1. epilepsy
2. fever
3. partial
4. generalized
5. clonic
6. tonic
7. absence
8. status epilepticus
9. CNS, GI tract
10. lorazepam
11. lamotrigine
12. levetiracetam
13. oxcarbazepine
14. topiramate
15. valproic acid
16. zonisamide
17. phenytoin
18. phenytoin
19. oxcarbazepine, carbamazepine
20. ethosuximide

REVIEW QUESTIONS
1. b   2. a   3. d   4. c   5. c   6. b   7. c   8. b
9. a   10. c

Chapter 12

MATCHING
1. h   2. e   3. g   4. a   5. b   6. c   7. f   8. d

TRUE OR FALSE
1. t   2. f   3. t   4. t   5. f   6. t   7. f   8. t
9. f   10. t

SHORT ANSWER
1. Destruction or degenerative changes in dopamine-producing nerve cells
2. Control symptoms, maintain functional ability in activities of daily living, minimize adverse drug effects, and slow disease progression
3. Better control of symptoms, reduced dosage of individual drugs
4. Increases the effects of the anticholinergic drug
5. Anorexia, nausea and vomiting, orthostatic hypotension, cardiac dysrhythmias, dyskinesia, CNS stimulation (restlessness, agitation, confusion, and delirium), abrupt swings in motor function

REVIEW QUESTIONS
1. b   2. a   3. c   4. b   5. a   6. a   7. b   8. d
9. c   10. a

Chapter 13

SHORT ANSWER
1. Neurological and musculoskeletal disorders, muscle spasms and cramps, spinal cord injury, and multiple sclerosis
2. Cause CNS depression; use cautiously in clients with impaired renal function, hepatic or respiratory depression, and those who must be alert for daily function.
3. To relieve pain, muscle spasm, and spasticity without impairing the ability to perform self-care activities of daily living
4. Anticholinergic effects (eg, dry mouth, constipation, urinary retention, tachycardia), drowsiness and dizziness
5. Deficient knowledge: safe use of skeletal muscle relaxants (SMR); Risk of injury: sedation and dizziness related to SMR

FILL IN THE BLANK
1. dantrolene
2. carisoprodol
3. baclofen
4. cyclobenzaprine
5. metaxalone
6. methocarbamol
7. orphenadrine
8. cyclobenzaprine
9. metaxalone, tizanidine
10. dantrolene
11. baclofen
12. diazepam
13. methocarbamol
14. dantrolene
15. tizanidine

REVIEW QUESTIONS
1. c   2. a   3. b   4. a   5. c   6. b   7. a   8. b
9. b   10. c

Chapter 14

DEFINITIONS
1. State of profound central nervous system depression with complete loss of sensation and consciousness, pain perception, and memory
2. Hypnosis, analgesia, and muscle relaxation
3. Loss of sensation and motor activity in localized areas of the body
4. Involves applying a local anesthetic to skin or mucous membranes
5. Injecting anesthetic solution into the area of a large nerve trunk or nerve plexus at some access point along the course of a nerve distant from the area to be anesthetized

TRUE OR FALSE
1. t   2. f   3. t   4. t   5. f   6. f   7. t   8. t
9. t   10. f

MATCHING
1. b   2. e   3. g   4. c   5. h   6. i   7. a   8. j
9. f   10. d

REVIEW QUESTIONS
1. b   2. a   3. c   4. b   5. d   6. c   7. a   8. c
9. d   10. a

Chapter 15

DEFINITIONS
1. Self-administration of a drug for prolonged periods producing physical or psychological dependence
2. A craving for a drug with unsuccessful attempts to decrease its use; compulsive drug-seeking behavior
3. Feelings of satisfaction and pleasure from taking a drug
4. Physiologic adaptation to chronic use of a drug so that unpleasant symptoms occur when the drug is stopped
5. When the body adjusts to drugs so that higher doses are needed to achieve feelings of pleasure

SHORT ANSWER
1. Anxiety, tremors, muscle twitching, weakness, dizziness, distorted visual perceptions, N & V, insomnia, nightmares, tachycardia, weight loss, postural hypotension, tonic/clonic seizures, delirium, convulsions
2. Agitation, anxiety, tremors, sweating, nausea, tachycardia, fever, hyperreflexia, postural hypotension, convulsions, delirium
3. Sympathetic nervous system overactivity
4. Agitation, hyperactivity, psychosis, cardiac dysrhythmias
5. Anxiety, irritability, difficulty concentrating, restlessness, headache, increased appetite, weight gain, sleep disturbances

TRUE OR FALSE
1. t   2. f   3. t   4. t   5. f   6. t   7. f   8. t
9. t   10. t

MATCHING
1. j   2. f   3. i   4. g   5. a   6. h   7. c   8. e
9. d   10. b

REVIEW QUESTIONS
1. c   2. a   3. b   4. b   5. d   6. a   7. b   8. d
9. a   10. c

Chapter 16

FILL IN THE BLANK
1. narcolepsy
2. amphetamines
3. caffeine
4. Ritalin
5. modafinil
6. caffeine
7. No-Doz
8. doxapram
9. modafinil
10. theophylline

SHORT ANSWER
Espresso—120 mg
Iced tea—70 mg
Mr. Pibb—57 mg
Mountain Dew—54 mg
Instant tea—50 mg
Coke—45 mg
Diet Pepsi—38 mg

FILL IN THE CHART

Drug	Narcolepsy	ADHD
Amphetamine	x	x
Dexedrine	x	x
Provigil	x	
Adderall	x	x
Desoxyn		x
Focalin		x
Ritalin	x	x

REVIEW QUESTIONS
1. a   2. d   3. b   4. c   5. a   6. d   7. a   8. b
9. a   10. c

Chapter 17

MATCHING
1. j   2. i   3. g   4. c   5. d   6. h   7. f   8. b
9. e   10. a

FILL IN THE BLANK
1. afferent
2. parasympathetic
3. alpha-1
4. peripheral
5. preganglionic
6. epinephrine
7. efferent
8. ganglia
9. sympathetic
10. norepinephrine

REVIEW QUESTIONS
1. b   2. c   3. b   4. c   5. d   6. b   7. d   8. a
9. c   10. a

Chapter 18

FILL IN THE CHART

Alpha and beta activity	Alpha activity	Beta activity
dopamine (Intropin)	metaraminol (Aramine)	albuterol (Proventil)
epinephrine (Adrenalin)	oxymetazoline hydrochloride (Afrin)	terbutaline (Brethine)
ephedrine (Efedron)	phenylephrine (Neo-Synephrine)	isoproterenol (Isuprel)
norepinephrine (Levophed)	tetrahydrozoline hydrochloride (Visine)	dobutamine (Dobutrex)
pseudoephedrine (Sudafed)	tuaminoheptane (Tuamine)	isoetharine (Bronkosol)

MATCHING
1. e   2. g   3. g   4. e   5. j and c   6. e, f, and g
7. g   8. a, c, and j 9. e   10. a

TRUE OR FALSE
1. f   2. t   3. f   4. f   5. t   6. f   7. t   8. f
9. t   10. t

REVIEW QUESTIONS
1. a   2. c   3. b   4. a   5. c   6. d   7. b   8. b
9. c   10. c

Chapter 19

SHORT ANSWER
1. Decreases urinary retention and improves urine flow by inhibiting contraction of muscle in the prostate and urinary bladder
2. Decrease in heart rate, cardiac output, blood pressure, and aqueous humor in the eye, and bronchoconstriction
3. To suppress pathologic stimulation, not the normal physiologic response to activity, stress, and other stimuli
4. Drugs combine with alpha-1 and beta-1 and -2 in peripheral tissues and prevent adrenergic effects
5. Inhibits release of norepinephrine in the brain, decreasing effects of sympathetic nervous system, which leads to a decrease in blood pressure

FILL IN THE CHART

Drug	Angina	Myocardial infarction	Dysrhythmia	Hypertension	Glaucoma	Migraine
atenolol	x	x		x		
metoprolol	x	x		x		
nadolol	x					
propranolol	x	x	x	x		x
acebutolol			x	x		
esmolol			x			
sotalol			x			
timolol		x		x	x	
betaxolol				x	x	
carteolol				x	x	
levobunolol						
metipranolol						

REVIEW QUESTIONS

1. b 2. b 3. a 4. c 5. a 6. d 7. b 8. a
9. c 10. a

BETA-ADRENERGIC BLOCKING DRUG ACTIONS DIAGRAM

1. Epinephrine and norepinephrine
2. Beta-adrenergic blocking drug
3. Nerve endings
4. Receptor site on cell surface
5. Myocardial or other tissue cells

Chapter 20

FILL IN THE BLANK

1. parasympathetic
2. nicotinic
3. glaucoma
4. bethanechol
5. tacrine, donepezil, rivastigmine
6. neostigmine
7. edrophonium
8. physostigmine salicylate
9. pyridostigmine
10. donepezil
11. rivastigmine
12. tacrine
13. pyridostigmine
14. physostigmine
15. atropine

TRUE OR FALSE

1. t 2. f 3. t 4. f 5. t 6. f 7. t 8. t
9. f 10. t

REVIEW QUESTIONS

1. b 2. d 3. d 4. a 5. c 6. a 7. d 8. b
9. b 10. c

Chapter 21

MATCHING

1. d 2. a 3. g 4. h 5. f 6. e 7. c 8. b
9. i 10. j

SHORT ANSWER

1. Drugs occupy receptor sites at parasympathetic nerve ending, which leaves fewer receptors free to respond to acetylcholine
2. Stimulation followed by depression of the CNS; decreased cardiovascular response; bronchodilation, and decreased respiratory tract secretions; antispasmodic effects in gastrointestinal tract (decreased muscle tone and motility); and mydriasis in the eye
3. To prevent vagal stimulation and potential bradycardia, hypotension, and cardiac arrest

4. To decrease the spasm-producing effects of the opioid analgesic
5. Hyperthermia—hot, dry, flushed skin; dry mouth; mydriasis; delirium; tachycardia; ileus and urinary retention
6. Tertiary amines—excreted in urine; quaternary amines—excreted in feces
7. Causes secretions to thicken and form mucus plugs in airways
8. Have been associated with behavioral disturbances and psychotic reactions
9. Blurred vision, confusion, heat stroke, constipation, urinary retention, hallucinations
10. Dilation of blood vessels in the neck

REVIEW QUESTIONS

1. c 2. a 3. b 4. a 5. c 6. d 7. a 8. b
9. c 10. d

Chapter 22

TRUE OR FALSE

1. f 2. f 3. t 4. t 5. f 6. t 7. f 8. t
9. t 10. t

FILL IN THE BLANK

1. chemical messengers
2. erythropoietin
3. cytokines
4. hypothalamus
5. ACTH, cortisol, growth hormone

SHORT ANSWER

1. Hypothalamus, pituitary, thyroid, parathyroids, pancreas, adrenals, ovaries, and testes
2. Metabolism of nutrients and water, reproduction, growth and development, adapting to changes in internal and external environment
3. Ovarian estrogen—promotes maturation of ovarian follicles, stimulates growth and cyclic changes on the endometrial lining of the uterus, stimulates hypothalamic-pituitary system to regulate its own secretion
4. Water-soluble, protein-derived hormones are inactivated by enzymes mainly in the liver and kidneys and excreted in bile or urine. Lipid-soluble steroid and thyroid hormones are conjugated in the liver to inactive forms and then excreted in bile or urine.

REVIEW QUESTIONS

1. d 2. a 3. b 4. c 5. c 6. b 7. a 8. b
9. d 10. a

Chapter 23

MATCHING

1. g   2. c   3. j   4. b   5. d   6. f   7. e   8. i
9. a   10. h

TRUE OR FALSE

1. t   2. f   3. t   4. f   5. t   6. f   7. t   8. f
9. t   10. t

FILL IN THE BLANK

1. thyrotropin-releasing hormone
2. gonadotropin-releasing hormone
3. follicle-stimulating hormone
4. luteinizing hormone
5. prolactin-inhibitory factor
6. adrenocorticotropic hormone
7. thyrotropin releasing hormone
8. corticotropin-releasing hormone
9. antidiuretic hormone
10. corticotropin-releasing factor

REVIEW QUESTIONS

1. a   2. b   3. c   4. d   5. a   6. a   7. b   8. c
9. b   10. c

Chapter 24

FILL IN THE BLANK

1. fungal
2. glucocorticoids
3. aldosterone
4. hydrocortisone
5. prednisolone
6. mineralocorticoids
7. antacids
8. Entocort EC
9. androgens
10. inhaled

TRUE OR FALSE

1. t   2. t   3. f   4. f   5. t   6. f   7. t   8. t
9. f   10. f

SHORT ANSWER

1. Stimuli cause the hypothalamus to secrete corticotropin, which in turn stimulates the adrenal cortex to secrete corticosteroids
2. Causes growth retardation even when used in small doses and administered by inhalation.
3. Decreasing salt intake may help decrease swelling; eating foods high in potassium may help prevent potassium loss; vitamin D (meats and dairy products) may help or prevent osteoporosis; vitamin C may help prevent excessive bruising.
4. Betamethasone or dexamethasone
5. Predisone can be taken orally and is inexpensive.

REVIEW QUESTIONS

1. b   2. c   3. b   4. c   5. c   6. b   7. a   8. d
9. b   10. a

Chapter 25

FILL IN THE BLANK

1. iodine, tyrosine
2. simple goiter
3. levothyroxine
4. protein
5. levothyroxine
6. thioamide
7. iodine
8. liothyronine
9. TSH
10. intracellular protein synthesis

MATCHING

1. f   2. j   3. a   4. d   5. h   6. i   7. g   8. c
9. e   10. b

TRUE OR FALSE

1. f   2. t   3. t   4. f   5. t   6. f   7. f   8. t
9. f   10. t

REVIEW QUESTIONS

1. a   2. a   3. c   4. c   5. c   6. c   7. a   8. b
9. d   10. a

Chapter 26

FILL IN THE BLANK

1. parathyroid hormone, calcitonin, vitamin D
2. calcitonin
3. hypercalcemia
4. Vitamin D
5. calcitonin
6. calcitonin-human
7. raloxifene
8. tamoxifen
9. Tums
10. etidronate

SHORT ANSWER

1. Hypocalcemia, hypercalcemia, osteoporosis, Paget's disease, bone breakdown associated with breast cancer and multiple myeloma
2. Drugs are poorly absorbed from intestinal tract and must be taken on an empty stomach with water at least 30 minutes before any other fluid, food, or medication. The drugs are not metabolized. The drug bound to bone is slowly released into the bloodstream. Most of the drug that is not bound to bone is excreted in the urine.

3. By inhibiting bone resorption
4. Cell membrane permeability and function; nerve cell excitability and transmission of impulses; contraction of cardiac, skeletal, and smooth muscle; conduction of electrical impulses in the heart; hormone secretion; and enzyme activity
5. It is required for cell reproduction and body growth. It combines with fatty acids to form phospholipids, which are components of all cell membranes; helps maintain acid-base balance; is necessary for cellular use of glucose and production of energy; and is necessary for proper function of several B vitamins.

FILL IN THE CHART

Category	Calcium requirement
Normal adults	1000 mg/daily
Growing children	1200 mg/daily
Pregnant women	1200 mg/daily
Lactating women	1200 mg/daily
Postmenopausal women	1500 mg/daily

REVIEW QUESTIONS
1. b   2. d   3. c   4. b   5. b   6. c   7. a   8. d
9. a   10. c

Chapter 27

MATCHING
1. e   2. c   3. d   4. g   5. h   6. j   7. i   8. f
9. a   10. b

TRUE OR FALSE
1. t   2. f   3. t   4. f   5. f   6. t   7. t   8. f
9. t   10. t   11. f   12. t   13. f   14. f   15. f   16. f
17. t   18. t   19. f   20. t

FILL IN THE CHART

Drug	Classification	Onset of action	Peak	Duration	Special considerations
metformin (Glucophage)	biguanide		1–3 hours		older adults at risk for lactic acidosis
acarbose (Precose)	alpha-glucosidase inhibitor		70 minutes		taken with first bite of every meal
glipizide (Glucotrol)	sulfonylurea	1–1½ hours		10–16 hours	take 30 minutes before first meal
glimepiride (Amaryl)	sulfonylurea	1 hour	2–3 hours		give with breakfast or first main meal
pioglitazone (Actos)	glitazone	rapid absorption	2 hours	24 hours	administer without regard to food; increases effects of insulin
repaglinide (Prandin)	meglitinide	30 minutes	1 hour	3–4 hours	administer within 30 minutes of a meal

FILL IN THE CHART

Type	Onset	Peak	Duration
Regular Iletin II	½–1 hour	2–3 hours	5–7 hours
NPH	1–1½ hours	8–12 hours	18–24 hours
Humalog	15 minutes	½–1½ hours	6–8 hours
Humulin N	1–1½ hours	8–12 hours	18–24 hours
Lente I	1–2 hours	8–12 hours	18–24 hours
Ultralente	4–8 hours	10–30 hours	36 hours
Novolin R	½–1 hour	2–3 hours	5–7 hours

REVIEW QUESTIONS
1. c   2. a   3. b   4. d   5. b   6. d   7. b   8. d
9. b   10. a

Chapter 28

TRUE OR FALSE
1. t   2. t   3. f   4. f   5. f   6. t   7. t   8. t
9. f   10. f

SHORT ANSWER
1. Promotes growth in tissues related to reproduction and sexual characteristics
2. To prevent endometrial cancer
3. Pregnancy, thromboembolic disorders, suspected breast or genital tissues cancer, undiagnosed vaginal or uterine bleeding, fibroid tumors of the uterus, stroke victims, heart disease, family history of breast cancer
4. Inhibits hypothalamic secretion of gonadotropin-releasing hormone, which inhibits pituitary secretion of FSH and LH, which stops ovulation; produces mucus that resists penetration of sperm into upper reproductive tract; interferes with endometrial maturation and reception of ova that are released and fertilized
5. Has been associated with vaginal cancer in female offspring and possible harmful effects on the male

FILL IN THE BLANK
1. progesterone
2. liver
3. estrogen
4. progesterone
5. ethinyl estradiol
6. black cohosh
7. Preven
8. Estraderm
9. Cenestin
10. progestins

REVIEW QUESTIONS
1. c   2. b   3. d   4. a   5. a   6. d   7. b   8. b
9. d   10. b

Chapter 29

SHORT ANSWER
1. Testes, ovaries, and adrenal cortices
2. Development of male sexual characteristics; reproduction; and metabolism
3. Because of abuse potential
4. Hypertension, decreased HDL, increased LDL, benign and malignant neoplasms, aggression, hostility, combativeness, decreased testicular function, amenorrhea, acne

FILL IN THE BLANK
1. cholesterol
2. estrogens
3. testosterone
4. Testoderm
5. scrotum
6. danazol
7. danazol
8. liver
9. Leydig's
10. anabolism, catabolism

REVIEW QUESTIONS
1. b   2. b   3. b   4. b   5. a   6. d   7. a   8. b
9. a   10. c

Chapter 30

MATCHING
1. e   2. i   3. d   4. a   5. h   6. j   7. c   8. b
9. f   10. g

TRUE OR FALSE
1. f   2. f   3. t   4. t   5. t   6. f   7. f   8. t
9. t   10. f

FILL IN THE CHART

Formula	Nutritional value	Uses
Enfamil	Complete	Alone for bottle, supplement for breast-fed babies
Lofenalac	Contains less phenylalanine	Infants and children with phenylketonuria
Pregestimil	Contains easily digested protein, fat and carbohydrates	Infants with severe malabsorption disorders
Prosobee	Milk free, contains soy and protein, 20 cal/oz	Infants who are allergic to milk
Isocal	Complete	Used as only source of nutrients or as a supplement
MCT Oil	Complete, contains an easily digested form of fat	Clients with fat malabsorption problems
Vivonex	Complete, high protein	Clients with severe burns, trauma, or sepsis
Amin-Aid	Provides amino acids, carbohydrates, and some electrolytes	Clients with renal failure
Nutrivent	High in fat and low in carbohydrates	Clients with chronic obstructive pulmonary disease
Polycose	Oral supplement	Clients on protein, electrolyte, or fat-restricted diets
PediaSure	Complete	Children 1–6 years old

REVIEW QUESTIONS
1. b 2. a 3. c 4. a 5. a 6. c 7. a 8. c
9. b 10. a

Chapter 31

MATCHING
1. f 2. g 3. e 4. h 5. c 6. a 7. i 8. d
9. b 10. j

FILL IN THE BLANK
1. B_{12}
2. A, E
3. A
4. C
5. Folic acid, C
6. Niacin
7. A
8. E
9. Folic acid
10. Niacin

DEFINITIONS
1. Recommended amounts of vitamins and some minerals
2. Amount of nutrient estimated to meet the needs of almost all (98%) healthy persons in a specific age and sex group
3. Amount thought to be sufficient when there is not enough reliable scientific information to estimate an average requirement

4. Amount of a nutrient estimated to provide adequate intake in 50% of healthy persons in a specific group
5. Maximum intake considered unlikely to pose a health risk in almost all healthy persons in a specific group

REVIEW QUESTIONS
1. a 2. b 3. a 4. d 5. d 6. c 7. a 8. b
9. a 10. c

Chapter 32

FILL IN THE BLANK
1. minerals
2. electrolytes
3. acid-base
4. macronutrients
5. micronutrients, trace elements

MATCHING
1. g 2. i 3. f 4. e 5. h 6. c 7. b 8. d
9. j 10. a

FILL IN THE CHART

Imbalance	Cause	Signs and Symptoms
Hyperkalemia	excessive intake, renal insufficiency, burns, crushing injuries and acidosis	serum potassium level >5 mEq/L, muscle weakness, respiratory insufficiency, cardiotoxicity
Hypochloremia metabolic alkalosis	vomiting, diuretic drug therapy, diabetic ketoacidosis, excessive perspiration, or adrenocortical insufficiency	serum chloride <95 mEq/L; arterial blood pH >7.45; numbness of face and extremities; muscle spasms and tetany; slow, shallow respirations; dehydration, hypotension
Hypernatremia	deficiency of water in proportion to amount of sodium present, hyperaldosteronism, Cushing's disease	serum sodium >145 mEq/L, lethargy, disorientation, hyperactive reflexes, muscle rigidity, tremors, spasms, irritability, coma, cerebral hemorrhage, hypotension, fever, dry skin, increased BUN, increased urine specific gravity
Hyponatremia	sodium-restricted diets, excessive vomiting, diarrhea, perspiration, burns, Addison's disease	serum sodium <135 mEq/L, decreased BP, tachycardia, oliguria, increased BUN, headache, dizziness, weakness, lethargy, restlessness, confusion, anorexia, nausea and vomiting, abdominal cramps
Hypokalemia	vomiting; diarrhea; overuse of laxative, enemas, or diuretics; administration of insulin leading to movement of potassium out of cells	serum potassium < 3.5 mEq/L, ECG changes, dysrhythmias, postural hypotension, confusion, memory impairment, lethargy, apathy, drowsiness, irritability, muscle weakness, abdominal distention, constipation, polyuria, polydipsia, nocturia, hyperglycemia
Hyperchloremia metabolic acidosis	dehydration, deficient bicarbonate, hyperparathyroidism, respiratory alkalosis, increased intake of sodium chloride or ammonium chloride	serum chloride >103 mEq/L, arterial blood pH < 7.35, lethargy, stupor, disorientation and coma, increased rate and depth of respiration.
Hypomagnesemia	inadequate diet intake, alcoholism, losses from diarrhea, diuretic drugs, or diabetic acidosis	serum magnesium <1.5 mEq/L, confusion, restlessness, irritability, vertigo, ataxia, seizures, muscle tremors, generalized spasticity, tachycardia, decreased BP
Hypermagnesemia	renal failure, excessive intake of antacids or cathartics, over treatment of magnesium deficiency	serum magnesium >2.5 mEq/L, skeletal muscle weakness and paralysis, cardiac dysrhythmias, hypotension, respiratory insufficiency, drowsiness, lethargy, coma

REVIEW QUESTIONS

1. c   2. c   3. a   4. c   5. c   6. b   7. d   8. a
9. a   10. b

Chapter 33

MATCHING
1. j 2. a 3. i 4. d 5. g 6. b 7. h 8. c
9. f 10. e

FILL IN THE CHART

Bacteria pathogen	Gram-positive or gram-negative	Normal in body flora	Medical conditions
Escherichia coli	gram-negative	intestinal tract	urinary tract infection (UTI), pneumonia, sepsis
Enterococci	gram-positive	human intestines	nosocomial infections, endocarditis
Staphylococcus spp.	gram-positive	skin, upper respiratory tract	boils, carbuncles, burn and surgical wounds, abscesses
Bacteroides spp.	gram-negative	digestive, respiratory, genital tracts	intra-abdominal and pelvic abscesses, brain abscess, bacteremia
Klebsiella spp.	gram-negative	bowels, respiratory tract, urinary tract, burns, wounds, meninges, bloodstream	pneumonia, sepsis, bacteremia
Streptococcus spp.	gram-positive	throat and nasopharynx	UTI, pneumonia, sinusitis, otitis media, meningitis
Proteus spp.	gram-negative	intestinal tract	UTI, wound infections

SHORT ANSWER
1. Intact skin and mucous membranes, anti-infective secretions, mechanical movements, phagocytic cells, immune and inflammatory processes
2. Widespread use of antimicrobials, interrupted or inadequate treatment, type of bacteria, type of infection, condition of host, location or setting
3. Inhibition of bacterial wall synthesis, inhibition of protein synthesis, disruption of microbial cell membranes, inhibition of organism reproduction by interfering with nucleic acid, inhibition of cell metabolism and growth

REVIEW QUESTIONS
1. b 2. a 3. c 4. d 5. c 6. c 7. d 8. c
9. c 10. b

Chapter 34

SHORT ANSWER
1. Penicillins, cephalosporins, carbapenems, monobactams
2. Inhibit synthesis of bacterial cell walls by binding to proteins that produce defective cell walls, which causes intracellular contents to leak, destroying microorganisms
3. Protects the penicillin from destruction by the enzymes and extends the penicillin's antimicrobial activity
4. Because the drugs are chemically similar

5. Rash, hives, itching, severe diarrhea, shortness of breath, fever, sore throat, black tongue, bleeding

MATCHING
1. j 2. g 3. h 4. b 5. i 6. d 7. e 8. f
9. c 10. a

TRUE OR FALSE
1. t 2. f 3. f 4. t 5. f 6. t 7. t 8. t
9. f 10. f

REVIEW QUESTIONS
1. c 2. a 3. b 4. d 5. c 6. b 7. b 8. a
9. d 10. b

Chapter 35

FILL IN THE BLANK
1. negative
2. kidney, inner ear
3. penicillin
4. neomycin, kanamycin
5. paromomycin
6. neomycin,

7. creatinine clearance
8. negative
9. antacids
10. ofloxacin

TRUE OR FALSE
1. f   2. t   3. t   4. t   5. f   6. t   7. t   8. f
9. f   10. t

REVIEW QUESTIONS
1. b   2. d   3. a   4. b   5. b   6. a   7. a   8. b
9. a   10. a

Chapter 36

SHORT ANSWER
1. Uncomplicated urethral, endocervical or rectal infections; adjunctive therapy for pelvic inflammatory disease (PID) and STDs; long-term acne; substitution for penicillin; traveler's diarrhea; inhibit antidiuretic hormone
2. Inhibits microlial protein synthesis
3. Act as antimetabolites of para-aminobenzoic acid (PABA) required to produce folic acid. Causes formation of nonfunctional derivatives of folic acid. Halts multiplication of new bacteria but does not kill mature, fully formed bacteria.
4. Deposited in bones and teeth along with calcium. Can cause permanent brown coloring of tooth enamel
5. Assessment data, force fluids, appropriate cleansing after sexual intercourse, take all medication, and take as directed

TRUE OR FALSE
1. f   2. t   3. t   4. f   5. t   6. f   7. f   8. t
9. t   10. f

REVIEW QUESTIONS
1. d   2. d   3. a   4. b   5. a   6. b   7. b   8. c
9. b   10. c

Chapter 37

MATCHING
1. i   2. j   3. a   4. e   5. d   6. f   7. h   8. b
9. c   10. g

TRUE OR FALSE
1. t   2. f   3. t   4. t   5. f   6. t   7. f   8. t
9. f   10. t

REVIEW QUESTIONS
1. c   2. d   3. b   4. b   5. a   6. b   7. b   8. b
9. a   10. a

Chapter 38

SHORT ANSWER
1. Penetrates body cells and mycobacteria, kills actively growing intracellular and extracellular organisms, and inhibits growth of dormant organisms in macrophages and tuberculous lesions.
2. LTBI—mycobacteria is inactive but remains alive in the body. There are no symptoms and the infection does not spread to others. Will have a positive TB skin test. Can develop active TB later. Active—usually results from reactivation of latent infection. Will have persistent cough and productive sputum, chest pain, chill, fever, hemoptysis, night sweats, weight loss, weakness, lack of appetite. Will have positive skin test and abnormal chest x-ray.
3. An increase in drug-resistant infections
4. By performing and reading TB skin tests, tracking contacts, assessing clients/homes, etc., educating clients and families, administering prescribed drugs, and maintaining records.
5. Isoniazid, rifampin, pyrazinamide, ethambutol, and streptomycin

MATCHING
1. c   2. d   3. h   4. g   5. f   6. i   7. j   8. b
9. a   10. e

TRUE OR FALSE
1. f   2. t   3. t   4. f   5. f   6. t   7. t   8. t
9. f   10. t

REVIEW QUESTIONS
1. a   2. a   3. d   4. b   5. c   6. b   7. d   8. b
9. a   10. d

Chapter 39

FILL IN THE BLANK
1. parasites
2. viruses, antibodies
3. acyclovir, famciclovir, valacyclovir
4. acyclovir
5. famciclovir, valacyclovir
6. valgarniclovir, ganciclovir
7. granulocytopenia, thrombocytopenia
8. trifluridine, vidarabine
9. zidovudine
10. tenofovir
11. ritonavir
12. amprenavir
13. Kaletra
14. amantadine, rimantadine
15. ribavirin

SHORT ANSWER

1. Fever, headache, cough, malaise, muscle pain, nausea, vomiting, diarrhea, insomnia, photophobia, normal WBC
2. Nucleoside and nonnucleoside reverse transcriptase inhibitors, nucleotide reverse transcriptase inhibitors, protease inhibitors
3. Gastrointestinal upset—anorexia and nausea, CNS symptoms—nervousness, lightheadedness, difficulty concentrating
4. Because they decrease the serum level of antiviral agents
5. Inhibit viral reproduction but do not eliminate viruses from tissues

REVIEW QUESTIONS

1. b   2. b   3. d   4. a   5. c   6. b   7. a   8. d
9. a   10. b

Chapter 40

MATCHING

1. e   2. j   3. c   4. i   5. b   6. g   7. h   8. d
9. f   10. a   11. k   12. l   13. m   14. q   15. n   16. o
17. p   18. r   19. s   20. t

TRUE OR FALSE

1. t   2. f   3. t   4. f   5. t   6. t   7. f   8. t
9. f   10. t

REVIEW QUESTIONS

1. c   2. b   3. a   4. b   5. b   6. d   7. b   8. a
9. c   10. a

Chapter 41

MATCHING

1. c   2. b   3. m   4. n   5. l   6. a   7. d   8. o
9. k   10. h   11. g   12. i   13. e   14. f   15. j

REVIEW QUESTIONS

1. b   2. c   3. d   4. a   5. a   6. a   7. a   8. c
9. b   10. d

Chapter 42

FILL IN THE BLANK

1. cytokines
2. interferons
3. interleukins
4. immune system
5. intact skin
6. inflammation
7. chemotaxis
8. histocompatibility complex

9. passive immunity
10. antigens
11. antibodies
12. immune
13. granulocytes
14. neutrophils
15. eosinophils
16. basophils
17. T lymphocytes
18. autoimmune
19. allergic
20. humoral

REVIEW QUESTIONS

1. b   2. a   3. d   4. c   5. b   6. a   7. c   8. b
9. d   10. c

Chapter 43

TRUE OR FALSE

1. t   2. f   3. t   4. f   5. f   6. f   7. f   8. t
9. t   10. f   11. t   12. f   13. t   14. t   15. t   16. t
17. f   18. f   19. t   20. t   21. t   22. t   23. t   24. f
25. t

REVIEW QUESTIONS

1. c   2. b   3. a   4. a   5. d   6. d   7. a   8. d
9. b   10. c

Chapter 44

SHORT ANSWER

1. To restore normal function or increase the ability of the immune system to eliminate harmful invaders
2. Difficulty in maintaining effective dose levels over treatment periods of weeks or months; some of the drugs have a short half-life and require frequent administration; are very powerful and cause adverse effects
3. Produce enzymes that inhibit protein synthesis and degrade viral RNA
4. Stimulates the immune system and elicits a local inflammatory response
5. They are proteins that will be destroyed by digestive enzymes.

FILL IN THE BLANK

1. oprelvekin
2. interferons
3. darbepoetin alfa, epoetin
4. aldesleukin
5. filgrastim
6. interferon alfa-2b
7. Avonex
8. antineoplastic
9. corticosteroids
10. interferons

REVIEW QUESTIONS

1. d   2. d   3. b   4. a   5. b   6. d   7. c   8. a
9. b   10. a

Chapter 45

MATCHING

1. c   2. g   3. d   4. e   5. f   6. h   7. j   8. b
9. a   10. i

TRUE OR FALSE

1. t   2. f   3. t   4. f   5. t   6. t   7. t   8. f
9. f   10. t

REVIEW QUESTIONS

1. c   2. a   3. c   4. a   5. d   6. d   7. c   8. a
9. d   10. a

Chapter 46

MATCHING

1. e   2. h   3. b   4. f   5. j   6. a   7. d   8. g
9. c   10. i

SHORT ANSWER

1. 21%
2. 16 to 20 times/min
3. 500 mL
4. 6 to 10 times/hr
5. Cough, increased secretions, mucosal congestion, and bronchospasms

REVIEW QUESTIONS

1. b   2. c   3. a   4. d   5. b   6. c   7. d   8. a
9. b   10. d

RESPIRATORY SYSTEM DIAGRAM

1. b   2. a   3. d   4. c   5. g   6. e   7. f

Chapter 47

TRUE OR FALSE

1. f   2. t   3. t   4. f   5. t   6. f   7. t   8. f
9. f   10. f

FILL IN THE BLANK

1. formoterol, salmeterol
2. metaproterenol
3. terbutaline
4. ipratropium
5. theophylline
6. leukotrienes
7. zileuton
8. ipratropium
9. terbutaline
10. corticosteroid

REVIEW QUESTIONS

1. c   2. d   3. c   4. a   5. d   6. d   7. b   8. b
9. d   10. a

Chapter 48

SHORT ANSWER

1. Secretory granules of mast and basophils cells—mostly tissue of skin and mucosal surfaces of eye, nose, lungs, and GI tract
2. Response to certain stimuli (allergic reactions, cellular injury, and extreme cold)
3. Mainly on smooth muscle cells in blood vessels and the respiratory and GI tract
4. Contraction of smooth muscle in bronchi and bronchioles; stimulation of vagus nerve endings to produce reflex bronchoconstriction and cough; increase in permeability of veins and capillaries, which causes fluid to flow into subcutaneous tissues and form edema; increased secretions of mucous glands; stimulation of sensory peripheral nerve endings to cause pain and pruritus; dilation of capillaries in the skin to cause flushing
5. Increased secretion of gastric acid and pepsin; increased rate and force of myocardial contraction; decreased immunologic and inflammatory reactions

MATCHING

1. j   2. c   3. b   4. d   5. f   6. g   7. h   8. e
9. i   10. a

REVIEW QUESTIONS

1. c   2. a   3. c   4. a   5. b   6. b   7. a   8. d
9. b   10. a

Chapter 49

FILL IN THE BLANK

1. skin, environmental surfaces
2. 10
3. rhinovirus
4. 5
5. handwashing
6. rhinitis
7. medulla oblongata
8. rhinorrhea
9. mucolytics
10. viral

COMPLETE THE CHART

Drug	Antihistamine	Nasal decongestant	Analgesic	Antitussive	Expectorant
Sinutab, sinus, allergy	x	x	x		
TheraFlu, flu, cold, cough	x	x	x	x	
NyQuil, cold, flu	x	x	x	x	
Contact, day, night, cold, flu	x	x	x	x	
Advil, cold, sinus		x	x		
Actifed, cold, allergy	x	x			
Cheracol D, cough, liquid				x	x
Comtrex, cold, sinus	x	x	x		
Coricidin D, cold	x	x	x		

REVIEW QUESTIONS
1. a   2. d   3. a   4. b   5. c   6. a   7. b   8. a
9. a   10. b

Chapter 50

SHORT ANSWER
1. Carry oxygen, nutrients, hormones, antibodies, and other substances to all body cells; remove waste products of cell metabolism (carbon dioxide and others)
2. Muscular organ, functions as a two-sided pump, circulates 5 to 6 liters of blood through the body every minute
3. Maintains one-way flow of blood and prevents backflow
4. Artery to artery anastomoses, which dilate to supply blood to the heart when a major artery is occluded
5. Connect the arterial and venous portions of the circulation

MATCHING
1. c   2. g   3. h   4. f   5. j   6. d   7. e   8. i
9. b   10. a

REVIEW QUESTIONS
1. c   2. b   3. a   4. b   5. b   6. a   7. c   8. d
9. a   10. b

CARDIOVASCULAR DIAGRAM
1. Superior vena cava
2. Coronary arteries
3. Right atrium
4. Tricuspid valve
5. Inferior vena cava
6. Papillary muscle
7. Aorta
8. Pulmonary artery
9. Left atrium
10. Mitral valve
11. Chordae tendon
12. Left ventricle
13. Septum
14. Right ventricle

Chapter 51

DEFINITIONS
1. When the heart cannot pump enough blood to meet tissue needs for oxygen
2. A neurohormone that acts as a vasoconstrictor and may exert toxic effects on the heart, resulting in myocardial cell proliferation
3. Administration of a sufficient amount of digitalis to produce therapeutic effects

SHORT ANSWER
1. Blood clot formation and vasoconstriction that narrows the blood vessel lumen, which causes coronary artery disease and hypertension, leading to heart failure
2. An enzyme produced in the kidney that stimulates production of angiotensin II, a vasconstrictor. This increases resistance, which causes increased pressure inside the heart, increasing stress on the myocardial wall and causing ischemia.

TRUE OR FALSE

1. f   2. t   3. f   4. t   5. t   6. f   7. f   8. t
9. t   10. f   11. t   12. f   13. f   14. f   15. t

MATCHING

1. e   2. g   3. c   4. h   5. d   6. i   7. j   8. a
9. b   10. f

REVIEW QUESTIONS

1. b   2. a   3. a   4. c   5. c   6. a   7. b   8. b
9. b   10. a

3. sodium
4. excitability
5. absolute refractory
6. relative refractory
7. conductivity
8. disturbances
9. hypomagnesemia
10. atrial fibrillation
11. digoxin,
12. supraventricular tachydysrhythmias
13. ventricular
14. radio frequency catheter ablation, surgical procedures and pacing
15. hypoxia, ischemia, acid-base, or electrolyte imbalances

Chapter 52

FILL IN THE BLANK

1. sodium, calcium, potassium
2. calcium

FILL IN THE CHART

Drug	Dysrhythmia use	Classification	Therapeutic level	Adverse effects
lidocaine	serious ventricular dysrhythmias	sodium channel blocker	2 to 5 mcg/mL	hypersensitivity reactions, muscle twitching, convulsions
quinidine	supraventricular and ventricular dysrhythmias	sodium channel blocker	2 to 6 mcg/mL	hypersensitivity reactions, tinnitis, vomiting, diarrhea, vertigo, headache
verapamil	paroxysmal supraventricular tachydysrhythmia (PSVT), atrial fibrillation, and atrial flutter	calcium channel blocker	0.08 to 0.3 mcg/mL	constipation
amiodarone	ventricular tachycardia or ventricular fibrillation	potassium channel blocker	0.5 to 2.5 mcg/mL	hyper- and hypothyroidism, hypotension, CNS disturbances, myocardial depression, peripheral neuropathy, photosensitivity
disopyramide	ventricular tachycardia	sodium channel blocker	2 to 8 mcg/mL	hypotension, blurred vision, dry mouth, constipation

MATCHING

1. j   2. i   3. b   4. c   5. e   6. d   7. g   8. a
9. f   10. h

REVIEW QUESTIONS

1. c   2. d   3. a   4. a   5. c   6. b   7. a   8. c
9. d   10. a

CARDIAC ELECTROPHYSIOLOGY DIAGRAM, PART I

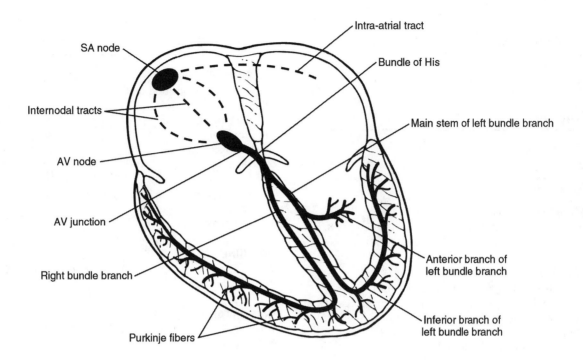

CARDIAC ELECTROPHYSIOLOGY DIAGRAM, PART II
1. SA node, AV node
2. AV node, bundle of His, right bundle branch, main stem of left bundle branch, anterior branch of left bundle branch, anterior branch of left bundle branch
3. SA node, AV node

DYSRHYTHMIA ANALYSIS
1. Supraventricular tachycardia, adenosine (Adenocard)
2. Atrial fibrillation, digoxin (Lanoxin)
3. Sinus bradycardia, atropine
4. Premature ventricular contractions, lidocaine (Xylocaine)

Chapter 53

SHORT ANSWER
1. Atherosclerotic plaque in coronary arteries and coronary vasospasms
2. Atherosclerotic plaque narrows the lumen, decreases elasticity, and impairs dilation of coronary arteries, resulting in impaired blood flow to the myocardium
3. Classic, variant, and unstable
4. Substernal chest pain that is constricting, squeezing, or suffocating in nature. Radiates to jaw, neck, shoulder down the left or both arms or to back. Lasts about 5 minutes or less.
5. To increase blood supply to the heart

6. Organic nitrates, beta-adrenergic blocking agents, and calcium channel blocking agents

MATCHING
1. c   2. g   3. e   4. d   5. b   6. j   7. f   8. h
9. a   10. i

TRUE OR FALSE
1. f   2. t   3. f   4. t   5. f   6. t   7. f   8. t
9. f   10. t

REVIEW QUESTIONS
1. d   2. b   3. a   4. a   5. b   6. a   7. b   8. b
9. a   10. d

Chapter 54

MATCHING
1. a   2. e   3. b   4. d   5. c   6. f

FILL IN THE BLANK
1. adrenergic
2. dopamine
3. epinephrine
4. isoproterenol
5. metaraminol
6. norepinephrine (Levophed)

7. dobutamine, dopamine
8. norepinephrine
9. dobutamine
10. acidosis

REVIEW QUESTIONS
1. c   2. a   3. b   4. c   5. b.   6. a   7. b   8. d.
9. a   10. b

Chapter 55

TRUE OR FALSE
1. f   2. t   3. t   4. f   5. t   6. t   7. f   8. t
9. t   10. t

MATCHING
1. g   2. j   3. c   4. d   5. i   6. h   7. e   8. b
9. f   10. a

DISCUSSION
1. Neural—involves the sympathetic nervous system (SNS); SNS neurons control heart rate and force of contraction, as well as muscle tone of blood vessels. When blood pressure is decreased, SNS produces secretions or epinephrine and norepinephrine, which causes constriction of blood vessels and increases rate and force of contraction, resulting in blood pressure increase
2. Hormonal—the renin-angiotensin-aldosterone (RAA) system is activated in response to decreased blood pressure and releases renin. Renin converts angiotensinogen to angiotensin I. Angiotensin-converting enzyme (ACE) acts on angiotensin I to produce angiotensin II. Angiotensin II strongly constricts blood vessels, increases peripheral resistance, and increases blood pressure. Vasopressin, the antidiuretic hormone, is released in response to the decreased blood pressure. It causes retention of body fluids and vasoconstriction, which increases blood pressure.
3. Vascular—endothelial cells that line blood vessels secrete substances that maintain a balance between vasoconstriction and vasodilation. The vasodilators (nitric oxide and prostacyclin) decrease vascular tone and blood pressure.

SHORT ANSWER
1. Decrease salt in diet, control weight and fat intake, exercise, and avoid smoking
2. Obesity, increased serum cholesterol and triglycerides, cigarette smoking, sedentary lifestyle, family history, African American race, adrenal disease, cardiovascular disorders, diabetes mellitus, oral contraceptives, and neurologic disorders

REVIEW QUESTIONS
1. c   2. d   3. a   4. c   5. b   6. c   7. d   8. a
9. d   10. b

Chapter 56

FILL IN THE BLANK
1. volume, composition, pH
2. nephron
3. glomerulus, tubule
4. proximal tubule
5. hydrogen ions
6. edema
7. convoluted
8. reabsorption
9. water
10. aldosterone

MATCHING
1. h   2. i   3. g   4. j   5. a   6. d   7. c   8. e
9. f   10. b

TRUE OR FALSE
1. f   2. f   3. t   4. t   5. f   6. f   7. t   8. t
9. t   10. t

REVIEW QUESTIONS
1. c   2. b   3. a   4. a   5. a   6. c   7. b   8. d
9. b   10. a

THE NEPHRON DIAGRAM
1. Efferent arteriole
2. Afferent arteriole
3. Bowman's capsule
4. Glomerulus
5. Distal tubule
6. Proximal tubule
7. Collecting tubule
8. Descending limb of Henle's loop
9. Ascending limb of Henle's loop
10. Henle's loop

Chapter 57

FILL IN THE BLANK
1. thrombosis
2. embolus
3. atherosclerosis
4. myocardial ischemia
5. homostasis

TRUE OR FALSE
1. t   2. f   3. f   4. t   5. f   6. t   7. t   8. f
9. t   10. f

FILL IN THE CHART

Drug	Increases	Decreases
acetaminophen	x	
griseofulvin		x
carbamazepine		x
tetracycline	x	
furosemide	x	
fluconazole	x	
rifampin		x
estrogen		x
aspirin	x	
quinidine	x	

REVIEW QUESTIONS
1. b   2. c   3. c   4. b   5. a   6. b   7. b   8. d
9. b   10. a

Chapter 58

FILL IN THE BLANK
1. cholesterol, phospholipids, triglycerides
2. lipoproteins
3. serum
4. triglyceride
5. lovastatin
6. fibrates
7. statin
8. gemfibrozil
9. fibrates, niacin
10. soy

FILL IN THE CHART

Blood lipid	Desired level	Borderline level	High level
Triglycerides	<150 mg/dL	150–199 mg/dL	200+ mg/dL
Total serum cholesterol	<200 mg/dL	200–239 mg/dL	240+ mg/dL
LDL cholesterol	<100 mg/dL	130–159 mg/dL	160+ mg/dL
HDL cholesterol	40–60 mg/dL	N/A	>60 mg/dL

TRUE OR FALSE
1. f   2. t   3. t   4. t   5. f   6. f   7. t   8. t
9. f   10. t

REVIEW QUESTIONS
1. a   2. a   3. c   4. b   5. d   6. a   7. b   8. c
9. b   10. b

Chapter 59

MATCHING
1. f   2. d   3. i   4. e   5. b   6. g   7. j   8. c
9. h   10. a

TRUE OR FALSE
1. f   2. f   3. t   4. f   5. f   6. f   7. t   8. t
9. t   10. f

REVIEW QUESTIONS
1. c   2. d   3. a   4. b   5. d   6. b   7. d   8. b
9. a   10. c

DIGESTIVE SYSTEM DIAGRAM
1. g   2. c   3. a   4. b   5. e   6. d   7. f

Chapter 60

TRUE OR FALSE
1. f   2. t   3. t   4. t   5. f   6. f   7. t   8. f
9. t   10. t

Chapter 61

MATCHING
1. b   2. c   3. d   4. a   5. c   6. a   7. d   8. c
9. b   10. a   11. d   12. e   13. c   14. d   15. c

FILL IN THE BLANK
1. stress
2. gastrin
3. aluminum, magnesium, calcium
4. bismuth
5. cimetidine
6. omeprazole (Prilosec)
7. misoprostol
8. sucralfate
9. omeprazole (Prilosec)
10. Mylanta, Maalox

MATCHING
1. d   2. a   3. h   4. c   5. i   6. g   7. e   8. j
9. b   10. f

REVIEW QUESTIONS
1. d   2. a   3. a   4. c   5. b   6. d   7. b   8. b
9. c   10. a

FILL IN THE CHART

Drug	Bulk-forming laxative	Surfactant laxative	Saline cathartic	Stimulant cathartic	Lubricant laxative
Mineral oil					x
Dulcolax				x	
GoLYTELY			x		
Citrucel	x				
Mitrolan	x				
Castor oil				x	
Metamucil	x				
Milk of magnesia			x		
Colace		x			
Dialose		x			

REVIEW QUESTIONS
1. c   2. b   3. b   4. c   5. c   6. b   7. a   8. a
9. d   10. c

Chapter 62

MATCHING

1. o   2. l   3. h   4. c   5. g   6. k   7. e   8. f
9. b   10. j   11. a   12. i   13. n   14. m   15. d

REVIEW QUESTIONS

1. b   2. c   3. d   4. a   5. b   6. a   7. d   8. b
9. a.   10. a

Chapter 63

FILL IN THE BLANK

1. medulla oblongata
2. prochlorperazine (Compazine), promethazine (Phenergan)
3. benzodiazepines
4. dronabinol (Marinol)
5. meclizine (Antivert)
6. phosphorated carbohydrate solution (Emetrol)
7. scopolamine
8. metoclopramide (Reglan)
9. dolasetron (Anzemet)
10. dexamethasone (Decadron)

TRUE OR FALSE

1. t   2. t   3. f.   4. f   5. f   6. t   7. t   8. t
9. t   10. f

REVIEW QUESTIONS

1. a   2. b   3. c   4. b   5. a   6. d   7. d   8. a
9. b   10. c

Chapter 64

TRUE OR FALSE

1. t   2. f   3. f   4. t   5. t   6. f   7. t   8. f
9. f   10. t

MATCHING

1. j   2. d   3. g   4. h   5. b   6. a   7. c   8. f
9. e   10. i

REVIEW QUESTIONS

1. c   2. b   3. b   4. d   5. b   6. a   7. d   8. a
9. c   10. d

CELL CYCLE DIAGRAM

1. Mitosis occurs
2. Resting phase
3. RNA and enzyme required for the production of DNA are developed
4. DNA is synthesized for chromosomes
5. RNA is synthesized and the mitotic spindle is formed
a. taxanes or taxoids
b. vinca alkaloids
c. steroids
d. alkylating agents
e. antibiotics
f. nitrosoureas
g. antimetabolites
h. podophyllotoxins

Chapter 65

MATCHING

1. a   2. g   3. e   4. i   5. b   6. d   7. j   8. c
9. f   10. h

TRUE OR FALSE

1. f   2. f   3. t   4. t   5. f   6. t   7. t   8. t
9. f   10. t

FILL IN THE BLANK

1. vitreous body
2. retina
3. optic disk
4. trifluridine (Viroptic)
5. natamycin (Natacyn)
6. topical beta blockers
7. glaucoma, cataracts
8. tropicamide, cyclopentolate
9. glaucoma
10. prostaglandin analogs

REVIEW QUESTIONS

1. c   2. d   3. c   4. b   5. b   6. d   7. b   8. a
9. c   10. c

ANATOMY OF THE EYE

1. Iris
2. Cornea
3. Pupil
4. Anterior chamber
5. Lens
6. Vitreous body
7. Retina
8. Choroid
9. Sclera
10. Optic disc
11. Optic nerve

Chapter 66

MATCHING
1. i   2. b   3. g   4. f   5. h   6. o   7. k   8. d
9. j   10. l   11. c   12. n   13. e   14. m   15. a

TRUE OR FALSE
1. f   2. t   3. t   4. f   5. f   6. t   7. f   8. f
9. t   10. t

REVIEW QUESTIONS
1. d   2. b   3. d   4. a   5. b   6. c   7. b   8. c
9. a   10. b

Chapter 67

TRUE OR FALSE
1. f   2. f   3. t   4. t   5. f   6. t   7. t   8. f
9. t   10. f   11. t   12. t   13. f   14. f   15. t

MATCHING
1. a   2. d   3. c   4. b   5. i   6. e   7. j   8. h
9. f   10. g

REVIEW QUESTIONS
1. b   2. c   3. b   4. b   5. b   6. c   7. d   8. b
9. a   10. d